Also by Callan Pinckney:

Callanetics
Callanetics for Your Back

CALLANETICS COUNTDOWN

30 DAYS TO A BEAUTIFUL BODY

THE FIRM, SHAPELY BODY YOU WANT IN ONLY MINUTES A DAY

CALLANETICS COUNTDOWN

30 DAYS TO A BEAUTIFUL BODY

THE FIRM, SHAPELY BODY YOU WANT IN ONLY MINUTES A DAY

CALLAN PINCKNEY

With Judie Bazerman
Photographs by Stuart M. Gross
Research and technical assistance by Nancy Gerard, OTR

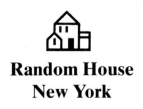

Random House
New York

All rights reserved under International and Pan-American Copyright Conventions.
Published in the United States by Random House, Inc., New York,
and simultaneously in Canada by Random House of Canada Limited, Toronto.

Published in Great Britain by Ebury Press

Library of Congress Cataloging-in-Publication Data
Pinckney, Callan.
    Callanetics countdown: thirty days to a beautiful body/by
Callan Pinckney with Judie Bazerman; photographs by Stuart M. Gross.
        p.   cm.
    ISBN 0-394-58613-1
    1. Exercise.   2. Stretching exercises.   3. Physical fitness.
    I. Bazerman, Judie.   II. Title.
    RA781.P5752   1990
    646.7'5—dc20   89-43548

Produced by The Miller Press, Inc.
Designed by Mary Moriarty

Manufactured in the United States of America

2 3 4 5 6 7 8 9

First Edition

Quality Printing and Binding By:
ARCATA GRAPHICS/KINGSPORT
Press and Roller Streets
Kingsport, TN 37662 U.S.A.

For Ebba Thomson and Mary Heriot . . .

Thank you for your kindness, support, and encouragement when I was a young child, and for your help when I was having such a difficult time finding my direction in life. But most of all, thank you for having faith in me. Both of you will always have a very special place in my heart.

Acknowledgments

Writing a book is a process that will never cease to amaze me. That said, I want to thank all the people who helped make this one possible, because it was not by any means a solo effort.

A very special thank-you goes out to Rebecca Saletan, my editor at Random House, for her invaluable assistance in organizing and reorganizing an incredible amount of material. Becky, I loved the way you jumped right in, literally getting down on the floor to do the exercises with me so that you would know and understand them firsthand.

Thanks also to Angela Miller, whose organizational abilities terrify me. Your feats in getting this book from manuscript stage to the printer may well have set a new world record for speed.

To my models—Lucy Jones, Will Trinkle, and Ann Whitney—thank you all so much! Even though you had not done Callanetics before, you were willing and eager to try everything. You succeeded in showing everyone just what a beginner can do. And, Lucy, I still can't believe you're sixty-two and the mother of six!

And finally, to my attorney, Marc Bailin, and my agent, Mitch Douglas, thank you for believing in me and for your continued support of all my whirlwind projects!

A Note of Warning

This program is intended for persons in good health. Before beginning this or any other exercise program, it is essential to obtain the approval and recommendations of your physician. It is suggested that you read through the text once to become familiar with the exercises before beginning the program.

If You Are Pregnant

If you are a woman in the first trimester of pregnancy, under no circumstances should you attempt the stomach exercises in this book. After the first trimester it may be safe for you to do these exercises gently, but clear this with your doctor first. Do not do any of these exercises unless your doctor has actually tried and experienced them personally before giving approval. Showing your doctor this book is not enough. Insist that he or she do the exercises to feel how deep the contractions are. At first glance, these exercises appear to be very easy, but in fact they may be too powerful to be performed during pregnancy.

A Message from Callan

You and I are about to embark on a journey, and it's my pleasure to welcome you as we begin to discover the wonderful machine that is your body. I am delighted that you have chosen *Callanetics Countdown* to help you make fitness and a beautiful body part of your life. I've walked all over the world, and I've learned that although every culture has its own idea of beauty, one trait all people share is that they care about the way they look and feel. This is a healthy trait. It's important to be happy with the way your body looks and feels—because how you feel about your body reflects how you feel about yourself.

The Callanetics Countdown can help you learn to love every part of your body. This series of exercises can tighten your muscles and get rid of all the hanging, dangling "goosh," as I love to call it, very quickly. Once that starts to happen, you'll find that you start to feel better about everything! But, remember, it's up to you—you must take responsibility. I can't change your life—but I hope I can help you change the way you think and feel about it.

Concentrate on what you are doing, and you will get amazing results. I know this not only because it happened to me, but also because thousands of people have told me about the well-being and happiness they have experienced through Callanetics. I have seen it alter countless lives in positive ways, and I believe that something that can do this must be shared. This is why I am so passionate about it. And once you start to see and feel the difference in your body, you will be, too.

C O N T

Acknowledgments • 9   A Note of Warning • 10   A Message from Callan • 11

Countdown to a Firmer, Shapelier You • 17

What Is Callanetics? • 18
What is a Beautiful Body? • 20
Making the Countdown a Part of Your Life • 23

Before You Begin • 25

How Long Is Thirty Days? • 25
How Many Problem Areas Can I Work? • 26
A Word about Format • 26
For the Best Results • 30
The Logistics • 31

P H A S E

DAYS 1 - 2 - 3 - 4
Page 33

WARM UPS • 34

The Underarm Tightener • 34
The Waist Away • 37
The Neck Stretch • 39
The Neck Roll • 41

THE STOMACH • 43

The Bent-Knee
Reach • 44
Single-Leg Raises • 47
Double-Leg Raises • 49
Both Legs Over • 51
Neck to the Side • 53
The Three-Quarter Neck
Relaxer • 55

LEGS AND INNER THIGHS • 56

Bend and Curl • 56
Plie and Balance • 59
Up and Over • 61
Hamstring Stretch • 63
The Standing Stretch • 65
The Inner-Thigh Tightener • 67

BUTTOCKS, HIPS, AND OUTER THIGHS • 69

Bringing Up the Rear • 70
Out to the Side • 72
Pelvic Circles • 74
The Pelvic Dip • 77
The Front-Thigh Stretch • 80
The Crossover • 82

P H A S E

DAYS 5 - 6 - 7 - 8 - 9
Page 85

WARM UPS • 86

The Underarm Tightener • 86
The Waist Away • 88
The Neck Stretch • 90
The Neck Roll • 91

THE STOMACH • 92

The Bent-Knee
Reach • 92
Single-Leg Raises • 94
Double-Leg Raises • 96
Both Legs Over • 97
Neck to the Side • 99
The Three-Quarter Neck
Relaxer • 100

LEGS AND INNER THIGHS • 101

Bend and Curl • 101
Plie and Balance • 103
Up and Over • 105
Hamstring Stretch • 107
The Standing Stretch • 109
The Inner-Thigh Tightener • 111

BUTTOCKS, HIPS, AND OUTER THIGHS • 112

Bringing Up the Rear • 112
Out to the Side • 114
Pelvic Circles • 116
The Pelvic Dip • 117
The Front-Thigh Stretch • 118
The Crossover • 119

E N T S

P H A S E III

D A Y S 1 0 - 1 1 - 1 2 - 1 3 - 1 4 - 1 5 - 1 6
Page 121

WARM UPS • 122

The Underarm Tightener • 122
The Waist Away • 123
The Neck Stretch • 125
The Neck Roll • 126

THE STOMACH • 127

The Bent-Knee
Reach • 127
Single-Leg Raises • 129
Double-Leg Raises • 130
Both Legs Over • 131
Neck to the Side • 132
The Three-Quarter Neck
Relaxer • 133

LEGS AND INNER THIGHS • 134

Bend and Curl • 134
Plie and Balance • 135
Up and Over • 136
Hamstring Stretch • 138
The Standing Stretch • 139
The Inner-Thigh Tightener • 140

BUTTOCKS, HIPS, AND OUTER THIGHS • 141

Bringing Up the Rear • 141
Out to the Side • 143
Pelvic Circles • 145
The Pelvic Dip • 146
The Front-Thigh Stretch • 148
The Crossover • 149

P H A S E IV

D A Y S 1 7 - 1 8 - 1 9 - 2 0 - 2 1 - 2 2 - 2 3 - 2 4 - 2 5 - 2 6 - 2 7 - 2 8 - 2 9 - 3 0
Page 151

WARM UPS • 152

The Underarm Tightener • 152
The Waist Away • 154
The Neck Stretch • 155
The Neck Roll • 156

THE STOMACH • 157

The Bent-Knee
Reach • 157
Single-Leg Raises • 159
Double-Leg Raises • 160
Both Legs Over • 161
Neck to the Side • 163
The Three-Quarter Neck
Relaxer • 164

LEGS AND INNER THIGHS • 165

Bend and Curl • 165
Plie and Balance • 167
Up and Over • 168
Hamstring Stretch • 170
The Standing Stretch • 171
The Inner-Thigh Tightener • 172

BUTTOCKS, HIPS, AND OUTER THIGHS • 173

Bringing Up the Rear • 173
Out to the Side • 174
Pelvic Circles • 175
The Pelvic Dip • 176
The Front-Thigh Stretch • 178
The Crossover • 179

Beyond the Countdown • 180

Maintenance • 180
The Winner Within • 181

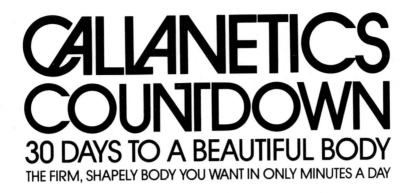

CALLANETICS COUNTDOWN

30 DAYS TO A BEAUTIFUL BODY

THE FIRM, SHAPELY BODY YOU WANT IN ONLY MINUTES A DAY

Countdown to a Firmer, Shapelier You

Ever since my first book caught on, people all over the world have been writing to ask me for a less time-consuming program. They'd like to be in better shape, but they can't seem to set aside time to do the regular one-hour Callanetics routine. I can understand that. It's a hectic, stressful world we live in—and I have the same problem! I've also received many letters asking me if there's a way to do only part of the Callanetics program—just the outer thighs and behind exercises, for example, or just the stomach exercises—to take care of problem areas quickly. It is because of these requests that I have written *Callanetics Countdown*. I believe that everyone, no matter how pressed for time, deserves to have the most beautiful body possible, and this book is my answer to all you busy, busy people.

You may be starting the Callanetics Countdown because you need a "quick fix." Perhaps you're going on vacation and suddenly realize that you will have to put on a bathing suit for the first time in months. Or perhaps you have a special occasion coming up and want to wear a slinky evening dress. Whatever your reasons for starting, I hope that after thirty days you will like what you see and how you feel enough to make health and fitness a permanent part of your lifestyle. My goal is to help you develop a new attitude—toward your body and your life!

You will find, as have many before you, that Callanetics is an ever-evolving process. No matter what your present age and condition, you'll soon find that your muscles are able to do things that seemed impossible the last time you tried. Working only twenty minutes a day, you'll find that the problem areas of your body will tighten and pull up. Within thirty days, you will see and feel quite a difference.

What Is Callanetics?

The essential principles of Callanetics have not changed. Instead, with the Countdown, I've developed a new way to get results.

How Callanetics Works

What all of my programs have in common is that they use series of exercises designed to work the body's largest muscles, very deeply, without making them bulky. It has been called the "no effort" exercise by some, but as anyone who has experienced Callanetics will tell you, it only looks effortless. It is not difficult, but you will feel your muscles working. As these large muscles become stronger, one experiences the exercises as working "deeper and deeper," as if in layers. By working these major muscles, you get fast results and the beautiful, springy body you deserve. And all of a sudden, movements you couldn't begin to do the first time will seem like child's play.

Moving the Callanetics Way

Callanetics has always stressed, and will always stress, tiny, delicate, precise movements, done in very slow motion—what I call *triple slow motion.* It is a very effective way to achieve a tighter, more youthful-looking body—and it's extremely safe. Once you have experienced the exercises, you will find that the emphasis is on techniques that prevent you from putting any strain on the lower back. These exercises actually alleviate pressure on the back, by stretching the spine at the same time that you are working the surrounding muscles.

Callanetics does not use any ballistic techniques, involving bouncing or jerking movements, which are a very easy way to pull a muscle.

The words my dictionary uses in defining *bounce* include *leap, jump, bound,* and *spring.* To me, all of these suggest sudden, quick, and large movements. You should *never, ever* bounce, or make any fast, jerky movements when doing Callanetics. It is very important that you understand that the movements are nothing like this at all. The movements in Callanetics are more like a pulse, which allows you to control the amount of force exerted on the muscle. The movements are tiny—one sixteenth to one quarter of an inch. Please get a ruler and take a good look at how small this is—most people are quite surprised. The movements are so subtle that they're almost just in your mind.

Long ago, I began to warn people against abusing their bodies with the awful jerking and swinging motions that are often erroneously equated with fitness. Research has proved me right, and it's very gratifying to see the tide turning and responsible people now starting to use slower motions that are gentler to the body. It also gives me a thrill when I hear that many instructors and doctors who keep up with the exercise world now recommend Callanetics. Unfortunately, though, some people continue to use "high impact" techniques, and for them the injury rate is still very high. Many programs now emphasize "low impact," but Callanetics has always been "no impact." Small, gentle motions teach you the wonderful feeling of using the body correctly. Once you achieve this awareness, you will be in control; the motions will not control you. That's how you'll learn what's going on in your body and how to listen to the signals it sends you. And that's how you prevent injury.

These tiny movements, however, perform many small miracles (some say large miracles). A conventional sit-up requires that you thrust your entire upper body off the floor, which means a terrific struggle against gravity. But most people's abdominal muscles are too weak to do this much work, so they compensate by involving other muscle groups—the back muscles (especially the delicate lower-back muscles) and even the legs. But the tiny, limited movements of the Callanetics stomach exercises, by contrast, give the abdominal muscles a task that *they and only they can perform, at the level they are capable of and no further.* As the muscles become stronger, they work at a deeper level. The same is true of the Callanetics exercises for other parts of the body.

Total Relaxation

Over and over in this book, you'll find me asking you to relax your body totally while doing an exercise. It's very difficult for people who haven't experienced Callanetics to understand what this means. Clearly, it is quite impossible to simultaneously contract and relax a muscle you are working—but that is not what I mean. What I'm asking you to do is not to forcefully tense your muscles—the ones you're working or any of the others. Tension—any more contraction than is necessary to perform the required movement—makes additional work for your muscles and exhausts them, keeping you from reaching the level you are capable of working at. The more you are able to relax, the more you'll discover you are able to do.

This state of relaxation is as much in the mind as it is in the body. People don't realize how tight their muscles get just from the stresses of everyday living and a lack of exercise. A body is not built to sit behind a desk all day. It needs to move! Recent studies have shown that muscle tone starts to deteriorate very quickly. It can begin to diminish in as little as two days. Just think about how you feel after you've been sick in bed for a while. You're wobbly! The muscles weaken because they haven't been used and they haven't been doing what they were designed for.

But people also don't realize how rigid and inflexible their overall outlook becomes, making them cranky and irritable as well as prone to tension headaches, muscle spasms, and a host of other aches and pains. Wouldn't it be wonderful if everyone could set aside a few moments every day to relax and meditate? But that's not very realistic for a lot of people. So here's an alternative: Use your exercise time to quiet your thoughts and get you into the habit of relaxing your body. Concentrating on your body will help you let go of everything else, and the more you relax, the faster the exercises will work, because there's no tension to work against. Just like taking a nap, relaxing replenishes your energy supply and clears out the cobwebs in your brain, helping you to look at things differently, more calmly. You'll learn to be in control and stay relaxed. You'll act instead of reacting, and that's really much healthier.

So if an exercise calls for you to lift your leg, for example, try to do so with a minimum of effort. Relax your toes, unlock your knees, try not to tense your shoulders. You'll discover that the gift of relaxation extends far beyond the immediate benefits of the exercise.

What Is a Beautiful Body?

There's no such thing as the Tooth Fairy, and there's no such thing as a perfect body. But the Callanetics Countdown can help you have a better body—a body you're proud of.

Having a beautiful body means different things to different people. One may be that you look good, in or out of clothes. Another—and I like this one especially—is that you spring out of bed in the morning, eager and ready to face the day, instead of feeling so tired that you tell yourself, "I'll just lie here for five more minutes." It means having an energy, an aliveness, that makes you ready to participate in life, not just drag yourself through it. Having a beautiful body does not mean conforming to a given set of measurements. But no matter what your body type or level of fitness, you will see improvements with the Callanetics Countdown. Dangling, "gooshy" skin doesn't look good on anyone, and no one has to live with it.

To get an idea of what Callanetics can do for you, start by identifying your body type. As you may already know, there are three basic types, called *somatotypes.*

Ectomorphs are naturally lean and tend to have rather angular features, long arms and legs, and narrow joints. They usually have a low ratio of body fat to muscle. Callanetics will help this type of body add definition and shape to the muscles.

Mesomorphs do not carry weight in any one particular place on the body. They are constitutionally strong, fairly compact, and usually have well-developed muscles. Their muscles, however, tend to droop and sag with underuse or age. Callanetics can tighten and "lift" them back into place.

Endomorphs are proportionally shorter-limbed than either of the other two. They tend to have wider hips, larger joints, and a higher ratio of body fat to muscle. They also tend to put on weight easily. Callanetics can reshape this body type by pulling in and tightening muscles. Weight will be carried better, and dieting may not be necessary.

Your body type is constant; that is, no amount of dieting or exercising will change it. It is determined by your genes. But the important thing to note here is that unworked, out-of-shape muscles don't belong to any of these body types. Personally, I don't care what type my body is, as long as it is tight, shapely, and powerful.

The good news is that Callanetics can affect most of the areas people consider "problems," like the size and shape of the legs, buttocks, hips, and waist, and the tightening of jiggly, slackened skin under the arms and elsewhere.

One of the first things that improves is posture. After doing the exercises for as little as one hour in total, you will actually see and feel a difference. This is because almost all the Callanetics exercises stretch the spine as the muscles contract. The neck area and the area between the shoulder blades gently loosen, and it becomes easier to pull back and stand more erect. The neck begins to look longer, and this can actually make you appear taller. Larger-framed people can look smaller because as the muscles get stronger and the body pulls up and in, body contours become sleek and tight. Even if you are already thin or work out regularly, Callanetics can enhance your appearance by tightening your muscles more than you dreamed.

Since the joints are supported and moved by groups of muscles on either side, strong muscles will make for strong joints, less susceptible to dislocation or ligament injuries. You will find that as your muscles get stronger, you can perform a wide variety of activities with a new-found ease and grace. Your step will get lighter. When teaching, I can gauge my students' progress as they arrive for classes. When they walk down the long hallway to enter the studio, I cannot see them—but I can certainly hear them. Beginners sound like a herd of buffalo as they stampede their way in. Several classes later, they are light as deer.

Fat: The Three-Letter Word

Callanetics has nothing to do with "burning fat," "losing fat," or "shifting fat." These are not expressions I use with Callanetics, but I do know this: They all have to do with weight loss, and that is something I have a definite opinion on.

If I had my way, you'd never get on another scale—or at least you'd limit it to your yearly checkup at the doctor's office. In most people, the problem is loose flesh, rather than excess weight. I am more interested in how the body looks than in numbers. With Callanetics, a lot of people can have a beautiful body without weight loss. However, if you decide you want to start a weight-loss program at the same time you start your Countdown program, Callanetics will make it look as if you've lost double the weight, because it pulls your muscles up and in so effectively.

Every time I say this, I think about one particular student of mine. She was quite a bit overweight, so she decided to combine Callanetics with dieting, and she succeeded in losing thirty-nine pounds. She looked wonderful. The people in her office were amazed. So many of them wondered how much weight she had lost that they decided to hold a contest. Twenty-two people entered. Do you know who won? No one! Everyone thought she had lost between eighty and eighty-five pounds!

In a healthy individual, about two pounds of every nine is fat. *Fat* seems to be a dirty word, but the truth is that everyone needs it. Especially in colder climates, fat is needed for insulation. It's also what keeps skin supple and smooth. Women have a naturally higher ratio of fat to muscle than men. Fat also tends to be distributed differently on women, accumulating around the abdomen, hips, and thighs. We women are often told that it's harder for us to get tighter in these areas because of this extra layer of fat. However, Callanetics is very effective at firming and tightening these areas in particular, because it works the muscles more deeply than regular exercises. By doing the Callanetics Countdown, you will find that you can tighten and firm almost any problem area, which is why I find the term *spot reducing* so confusing. The "experts" say there's no such thing. But if a given area gets tighter and more compact, then I say the results speak for themselves. Just the other day, I had a letter from a woman who said that through Callanetics she had lost *nine inches*, overall, on her legs. That sounds suspiciously like spot reducing to me, but does it really matter what we call it? That was a terribly happy lady I heard from.

Glorious Food

It is amazing to me how many people think they can starve themselves to beauty. Your body is a complex living thing, an intricate mechanism that needs fuel to function at peak efficiency. If you want a beautiful body, food, in the form of a nourishing, balanced diet, is the fuel your body needs. Callanetics will take care of your shape.

When I'm doing my Callanetics exercises regularly, I find that I don't even have to think about diet. Many of my students report that as Callanetics taught them to be more aware of their bodies, their attitudes toward food started to change. Exercise releases tension, and also causes the secretion of endorphins (the hormones that make you feel good) by the brain. Whatever the scientific explanation, many of my students have found that once they've undertaken a regular Callanetics program, junk food seems to lose its appeal. They no longer crave sugar. They start to watch and care about what they put into their bodies. Some cut down on fats, fried foods, sugar, and refined flour—and start to lose weight. They don't deprive themselves—they make healthy substitutions, like baked potatoes and whole-grain breads.

Some find that what works best is to eat very little past six o'clock at night. They also drink plenty of water. As any nutritionist will tell you, this is important to help your body flush out toxins. All report feeling more energized and alive. The key, I think, is moderation and healthful, whole foods—combined with exercise, of course!

One tip: I'm a chocolate addict—I even dream

about boxes of Godivas. But when I'm awake and the urge strikes, I take three or four deep sniffs of a candy bar—and the craving is gone.

Making the Countdown a Part of Your Life

The Callanetics Countdown is a highly flexible program, adaptable to almost any need or lifestyle. Whatever your profession, your age, your schedule, it can make your life healthier and more enjoyable.

The Callanetics Countdown is excellent for older people. Aging doesn't have to mean going over the hill as far as fitness and physique are concerned. So don't settle for less, and don't believe your own excuses: The Countdown can help you have the boundless energy you deserve, whatever your age.

It's true that every second of the day, gravity pulls your body down. As you age, everything tends to droop—even the end of your nose! I like to say that Callanetics defies gravity, because as you work to get your muscles strong, they lift, taking the skin with them. Everything rises, and is restored to a more youthful position. The muscles act like a natural girdle, holding you in and pulling you up.

As you age, your metabolism slows down, and consequently you don't burn calories as quickly. That is why people tend to put on weight over the years and find it so hard to take off "middle-age spread." However, Callanetics, unlike many other kinds of exercise, does not depend on burning calories for results, so everyone can get the same fast, safe benefits.

As described in the next chapter, the Callan-etics Countdown is easy to adapt to your specific pace and level of activity. Older people may find they need to take the progression more slowly, or stay at a given phase for an extended time. However you adapt the program, you'll find that it helps to combat the aches and stiffness of arthritis and may help prevent or slow the development of osteoporosis. Even if you're not yet old, you'll find that your circulation improves, your step is livelier, you're able to stand longer and walk further.

If you are a busy executive, the Callanetics Countdown is perfect for you. It doesn't require any special equipment, takes only twenty minutes a day, and can be done literally anywhere—in the office or even in a hotel room, when you're on a business trip. Once you become proficient at it, you can exercise and return phone calls at the same time, if you need to.

If you are a new mother and are like most women, you may feel that nature has stretched you in ways from which you may never recover! The Callanetics Countdown—especially the stomach exercises—can come to your rescue, and it's custom-made for your new schedule.

Babies tend to make their own schedules, with complete disregard for anyone else's. With the Callanetics Countdown, you can work around this. You can do your exercises while your baby naps or with him next to you on the floor, where you can keep an eye on him. You won't be waiting for a health club to open or for an exercise show to come on the television. You can make the best use of the time you have—even if it is the middle of the night! You may not feel that your body is at its best right at this moment, but think of what it's been through and be patient. With the Callanetics Countdown, you'll be able to work in the privacy of your home, and you'll see results very quickly.

It is usually suggested that you wait about six weeks after delivery before beginning any kind of exercise program, but you should, of course, check with your own doctor first. Once you begin, however, you will be amazed at how fast you will regain muscle tone, no matter what kind of condition you were in before your pregnancy. Begin slowly and take your time. Your ability will improve as your muscles become stronger, so it's very important to work at your own pace.

If you are nursing your baby, you may find that you are hungry all the time and eating much more than before. The Callanetics Countdown will help you keep your figure.

Fitness for All

It's important to learn good habits early. If you have children, you can start to teach them about their bodies at a very young age. It's important to convey that taking care of your body is fun! Most children are healthy and active enough not to have problem areas at a young age, and most have a natural flexibility and stretch easily. Therefore, I recommend introducing the Callanetics Countdown stretches when a child is around eight years old, although of course you should check with your family physician first. At this age, the child is alert enough to tune in to these body motions and feel what it's like to really use his or her muscles. It gives the child a

body awareness and a connection to self that, hopefully, will be retained as the child gets older. It is also an excellent way to encourage good posture.

Perhaps the nicest thing about Callanetics is that these exercises can be an opportunity for the family to do something together. Parents can lead their children, grandparents can help their grandchildren, and older children can guide their younger siblings. It gives you a chance to spend quality time together, doing something beneficial. If you like, you can turn on the television or pop in your favorite video, and the whole family can exercise and be entertained at the same time.

As you will see, the Callanetics Countdown is not just another exercise program. It can change your body, and it can transform your life! It draws upon the best elements of yoga, ballet, modern dance, t'ai chi, and belly dancing, as well as plain old common sense. The results you will see have been confirmed by my students over and over again. You will have more energy, feel better, move with more grace and ease, feel calmer—and get a tight, shapely body as a bonus! It won't take very long until you start to notice differences. Your legs will seem longer, your buttocks tighter and rounder, your thighs firmer, your stomach flatter, your waist smaller. Day by day, you will start to look a lot better to yourself. You will see yourself in a brand-new way, and you will start to appreciate your own special beauty—because no matter what your body looks like, it's going to look so much better with the Callanetics Countdown.

Before You Begin

Callanetics Countdown is a different type of exercise book. It offers a menu approach, in that you choose the area or areas you wish to work on, according to your needs. The thirty-day program is broken down into four phases, each progressively more advanced. Since your own development will proceed according to how strong your muscles are when you begin, there is no one "right way" for everyone to do the exercises. You must decide what is right for you. However, the more information you have, the more intelligent your choices will be. So let's begin with the obvious question.

How Long Is Thirty Days?

This book promises to help you handle your problem spots in thirty days. Does that mean a month? Four weeks? Thirty days in a row? The answer is up to you. To see results, you should practice your twenty-minute program thirty times. How you break it up depends on you and what your schedule allows. You can do it every day for thirty days. You can do it six days a week for five weeks, or five days a week for six weeks. It should be noted here that since everyone's body is different, only you can make the choice whether to exercise every day. Please note that these exercises, with their delicate, controlled movements, do not cause the wear and tear that weights, jerking, and the high-impact movements used in other kinds of exercise involve. It is therefore perfectly safe to do Callanetics every day. The main thing, however, is to do it, because the more often you do it, the faster you'll see results.

How Many Problem Areas Can I Work?

The problem areas of the body are broken down into three broad units:

1. the stomach
2. the legs (including inner thighs), and
3. the buttocks, hips, and outer thighs.

The twenty-minute program is based on doing the warm-up and one of these units. For example, suppose you want to flatten your stomach. Follow the thirty-day program for the stomach, which includes the warm-up and the appropriate exercises and stretches. Do these every time you exercise. If you have time and wish to work a second problem area, add the appropriate exercises and stretches (you needn't repeat the warm-up). Your program should take about ten to fifteen minutes longer with these added movements. As you get stronger, you'll find that you are able to move quickly from movement to movement with great control, and the program will take you less time.

A Word about Format

At the beginning of each exercise, you will find a description of the body areas the exercise works, and after the technique, a list of "*Don'ts*" that will help you avoid common mistakes.

At the end of each exercise segment, you will find the *Repetitions*. This will tell you how many repetitions of the exercise you are to do each time or how many counts to hold it for, and when to increase that number. If you find that you cannot do the required number of repetitions at one time, break it up into sets. For best results, you should try to complete the given number of repetitions. But safety comes first; never force yourself to do more than you are able. Switch from side to side if necessary to give the muscles a chance to rest between sets. If you find that you can do more than is required on a given day, you may want to increase the number of repetitions sooner than called for. If you feel you are strong enough, you can even go on to the next phase. You will then see results even faster.

It's important to follow the order of the program. Always start with the warm-up, then proceed with the exercises and stretches in the order they are given. Muscles are worked in a certain sequence so that fatigue does not come into play. You get better results this way.

The Callanetics warm-up is a bit different from the warm-ups you may be familiar with from other kinds of exercise. Because you won't be using a lot of force on your muscles during the Countdown, elaborate warm-ups aren't necessary. The exercises themselves both stretch and contract your muscles; in other words, they are their own warm-up. The *Warm-up* section at the beginning of each phase contains some easier stretching and contracting exercises that focus particularly on the neck, waist, and underarms. They'll get you psychologically as much as physically prepared to tackle the more challenging exercises that follow. Remember, this is a different type of exercise program, and consequently the warm-up is also different.

Callanetics is a total system of contractions and stretches. All the stretches have been designed to complement the particular exercises that follow. Doing the stretches will ensure

that you stretch the specific muscles you have been working. Stretching helps prevent common injuries such as tendon and ligament tears. It's also important because it lengthens the muscles after they have been contracted, and this prevents the development of bulky muscles. This system of doing contractions and gentle stretches together will get you the results you want, without injury.

Here are a few simple rules about stretching:

• Let your body tell you how far to stretch. Never compare what you can do to what another person can do when stretching. Some people's muscles have more flexibility, and may stretch more easily than others.

• Everybody is different, every day is different, and every time you stretch can be different, so don't expect your muscles to stretch the same way every day.

• Be gentle. Stretching the muscles also pulls the tendons and the connective tissue that surrounds your muscles. If not adequately stretched, the muscles can shorten, which may restrict your movement.

• Move in *triple slow motion* (see below).

There are certain terms I use throughout this book that you may not be familiar with.

Triple Slow Motion

To ensure that you control the motion, rather than the motion controlling you, I instruct you to perform the movements in *"triple slow motion."* To understand what this means, think of a movie or a television program being shown at a very slow speed. Now, slow your move-

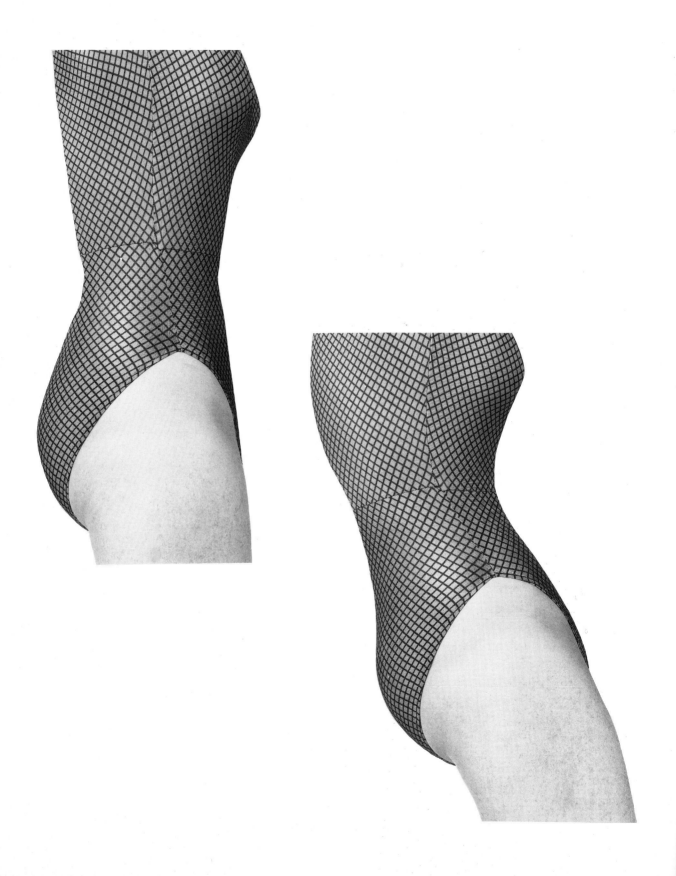

ments down *even more*, and you will reach triple slow motion. Working this way ensures that the muscles are treated with respect.

Curling Up the Pelvis

If there is one motion that is key to Callanetics, it is curling up the pelvis. The pelvis may be thought of as the link between the upper and lower body. There are no muscles used only for moving the pelvis, but its movement is controlled by the muscles of the legs and torso.

Tighten your buttocks, and in triple slow motion try to move, or "curl up," the pelvic area, as if you were trying to bring your pubic bone to your navel. This movement strengthens your abdominal, inner- and front-thigh, and buttock muscles, as well as your calves and feet, if you're standing. Once you have perfected the curl, you will feel the lower back stretching, and you will have more flexibility in your spine. As your muscles get stronger, you will be able to increase the degree of the curl.

Gaining freedom in the pelvic area is very important because it affects posture, balance, and alignment of the body. It also loosens the hip joints and allows for more fluid movements. This is one exercise that you can practice anywhere, anytime, even sitting down. Just remember, it does not mean sticking out your stomach or arching your lower back. It is a gentle rounding up, a beautiful flowing movement.

Breathing

When I started to teach, one of the first things I noticed was that people were trying to use complicated series of breathing maneuvers that had been required by other exercise instructors. They were concentrating on their breathing technique instead of on the exercises, and this usually had the effect of tensing the body just when it was supposed to be relaxed. This is the main reason that there are no special breathing instructions for Callanetics. What is taught in most exercise classes is really telling people to do what comes naturally: to inhale before a movement and exhale slowly during it. This is what will happen on its own, so I believe you should concentrate on your body movements rather than on your breathing. Breathe naturally—but remember to breathe! Many people actually forget to breathe when exercising.

Counting

Several of the exercises include instructions to "hold for a count of . . ." You should count "one thousand and one, one thousand and two," etc. If you count aloud, the added plus is that you'll be sure to breathe!

Pain

No one knows what is going on in your body but you. So try to listen for the signals it sends you. Your muscles will let you know if you are doing too much—or too little. For example, if you lose control and you start to tremble, you will know that the muscles are approaching fatigue. If this happens, stop that exercise for the day. Go to another exercise that works a different set of muscles and come back to the exercise that exhausted your muscles the next time you exercise. Just remember that different people have different discomfort thresholds, and what "hurts" one person may be bearable or pleasant to another. In any kind of activity, especially high-impact ones, the anticipation of pain often causes the body to tense more, which, in turn, can cause it to fix or stiffen, and this can lead to injury. Even though Callanetics is a very gentle form of exercise, it's important to remember to relax. Don't overexert your muscles or try to push your body into doing too much too soon. You can't make up for months or years of neglect in twenty minutes. Just work at your own pace and build up your strength gradually.

When you use a muscle in a new way or stretch one that hasn't been used in a while, you may feel a slight stiffness. Simply think of it as the muscle waking up. If you have to modify a movement to be comfortable, that is fine, as long as you are still working the muscle. What is *not* normal, in any type of exercise, is any sudden or sharp, stabbing pain—especially in the chest or arm, which can indicate angina—breathlessness, or dizziness. If this happens, stop. If the pain continues or gets worse, stop exercising and check with your doctor.

Soreness is a kind of discomfort that generally comes from muscles being exercised for the first time or from their being held in a state of tension. In some cases, for example in the neck and between the shoulder blades, what you are actually feeling, nine times out of ten, is the muscle being released from tension. It's important to keep exercising to fully undo the soreness and tightness.

For the Best Results

Some people may see more dramatic results than others, depending on their body type and the condition of their muscles when they begin. Here are a few miscellaneous tips to ensure that you get the most from the Countdown.

• Count repetitions carefully. Most people are stronger on one side and tend to favor it. I'll never forget the student who told me it was easier to work on her right so she did more repetitions on that side. She actually pulled in faster and became tighter on that one side! So, please, be aware and be sure to do the same number of repetitions on each side.

• If you develop any irritation when doing any exercises, such as redness from friction on the spine, place a small towel under you. Especially with the stomach exercises, some women find they have to undo their bras to avoid the hooks rubbing.

• If you are having trouble doing the exercises, take frequent breaks or rest periods. This helps to renourish your muscles. You will build up strength gradually, and can then decrease the number of breaks you have to take. Whatever you can do is right for you.

• Relax. Forcefully tensing your body wastes so much energy! Aside from exhausting you, the tension may actually cut off some of the blood supply. This can lead to sore muscles and the risk of spasm. Exercise is supposed to be fun! Remember, you're doing it *for* yourself, not *to* yourself.

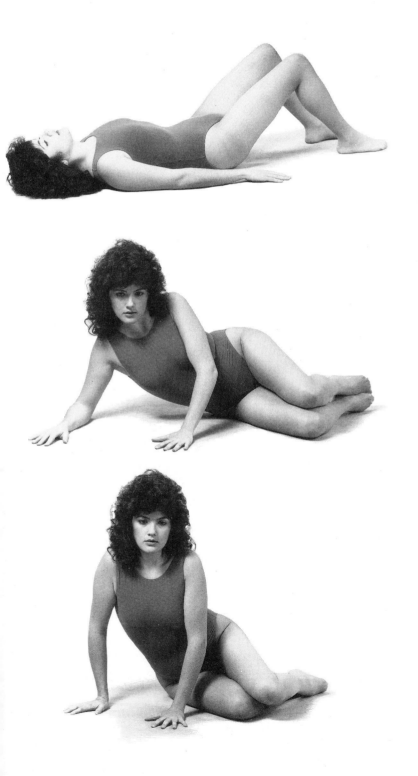

• There is a proper way to get up from the floor after doing exercises or stretches on your back. Roll onto your side and, with knees bent, push yourself up into a sitting position with your arms. Then stand up from there.

The Logistics

The Callanetics Countdown doesn't require special clothing. Wear whatever you're comfortable in, as long as it doesn't restrict movement. A lot of busy people who work in offices do Callanetics on a break or at lunchtime, in their street clothes! For most people, however, it's shorts, a T-shirt and socks, jogging suits, leotards, or the like. I don't recommend that you wear shoes, however, because they tend to be too heavy and put too much pressure on the joints, especially during the buttock exercises. Under no circumstances should you put weights on your feet or ankles. Your legs are heavy enough—any additional weight will be too much.

You can do the exercises just about anywhere you have

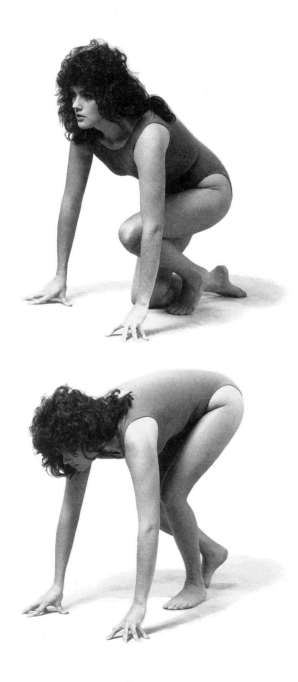

room to move about comfortably. You will need enough room to stretch out on the floor and fully extend your arms and legs, not much more. The room should be a comfortable temperature. Just remember, most people don't perspire doing Callanetics.

Some of the exercises call for a "barre." Be creative! You can use anything from the counter in your kitchen to the desk in your office. Use a chair, a sofa, a trunk, or even a filing cabinet. Just make sure that whatever you use is sturdy enough to support your weight. The individual instructions will tell you how high the "barre" needs to be for a given exercise.

Especially in the beginning, I don't recommend the use of music or any distraction. I would rather you put all your concentration into relaxing your body and performing the exercises. When there is music on, the natural tendency is to follow the beat, and you may begin to make certain movements too rapidly. Without it, you will have control and you can set your own pace.

You are now ready to put everything you've learned into action. It's time to start on your way to having the beautiful, strong, flexible body you've always secretly dreamed of!

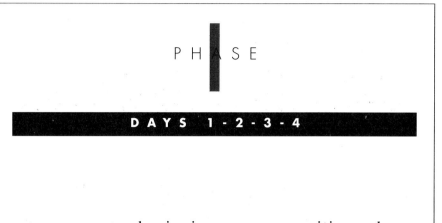

PHASE I

DAYS 1-2-3-4

You are beginning a very exciting adventure—you're about to discover your body! Take the time to read the directions carefully before you begin, and for the first few days concentrate on getting every detail right, even if the exercises seem awkward or difficult at first. Every movement is done for a reason, and this phase is the foundation for the three that follow. Once you start to teach your muscles to contract and stretch, it will be easier for you to progress in each phase.

You may find some of the exercises hard to do at first. This is because you are working your muscles very deeply, and you may not have used them in this manner for a long while—if ever. You may feel them working in places you don't expect. You'll probably feel a little sore, but this feeling should disappear as you become ready to move into Phase II. Just remember—the more you do these exercises, the more of a difference you'll see and the more "alive" your body will feel. In fact, after as little as two days of the Callanetics Countdown, your posture will already have improved and you will start to feel more energized. Enjoy the exciting new feeling.

WARM-UPS

The Underarm Tightener

It may not be anatomically proper, but *underarm* is the best term I've found to describe the under part of the upper arm—the part that tends to get loose and dangling. This exercise will help to banish underarm "goosh."

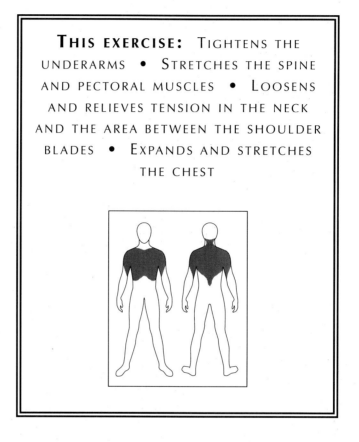

> **THIS EXERCISE:** TIGHTENS THE UNDERARMS • STRETCHES THE SPINE AND PECTORAL MUSCLES • LOOSENS AND RELIEVES TENSION IN THE NECK AND THE AREA BETWEEN THE SHOULDER BLADES • EXPANDS AND STRETCHES THE CHEST

❏ Sit on the edge of a chair or sofa, keeping your back straight and your feet resting comfortably on the floor. Do not lean back. Take your arms out to the sides. Try to keep them straight, at about shoulder level.

DON'TS

❏ **Do not jerk your arms back and forth.**

❏ **Do not arch your back or stick out your stomach.**

❏ **Do not lock your elbows.**

❏ **Do not tense your shoulders.**

❏ Slowly, turn your hands forward and over, so that the backs of your hands are facing the floor, and your palms and thumbs are facing upward.

❏ Leaning forward, very gently bring your arms back as far as you can, keeping them as straight as possible, as if you were trying to get the backs of your hands to touch. Try to hold your arms as high as possible as you take them back.

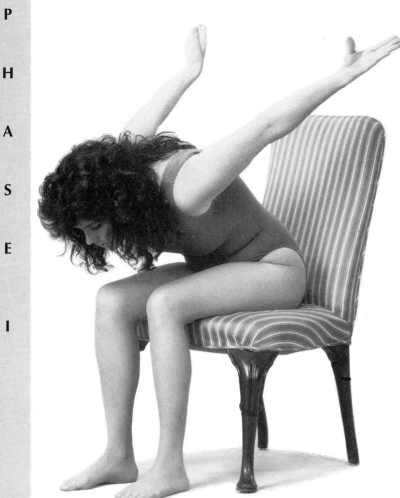

❑ Gently, in *triple slow motion*, move your arms one-sixteenth to one-quarter inch closer together and back, being very careful to avoid any jerky motions. After a few of these movements, gravity will pull your arms down and your head and shoulders forward from wherever you started. Be conscious of this, and try to return them to the proper position. You may not be able to keep your elbows entirely straight at first. (Some people are never able to straighten their arms fully; that's perfectly all right.)

❑ Upon completion, gently release your arms by bending your elbows and, in *triple slow motion,* return to the starting position.

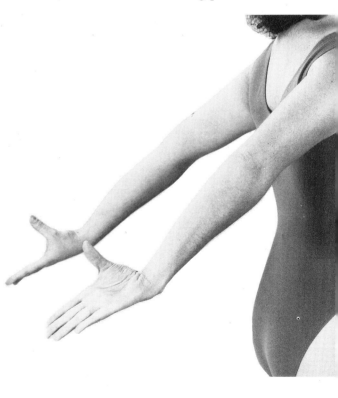

Repetitions						
DAY 1 **25**	DAY 2 **30**	DAY 3 **40**	DAY 4 **50**	5	6	7
8	9	10	11	12	13	14
15	16	17	18	19	20	21
22	23	24	25	26	27	28
29	30					

The Waist Away

An alternative to wearing cinchers and corsets!

THIS EXERCISE: STRETCHES THE WAIST, SPINE, BACK OF THE SHOULDERS, AND UNDERARM AREA
• REDUCES WAIST SIZE

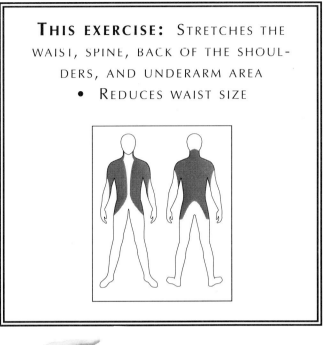

TECHNIQUE

❏ Sit up straight in an armchair and allow your left arm to rest on the arm of the chair. (If you don't have an armchair, simply rest your left palm beside you on the seat of the chair.) Keeping the spine straight, slowly stretch your right arm up to the ceiling, palm facing inward. Try to keep your arm by your ear. You should feel the stretch from your waist right up to your underarm. Now, stretch up and try to reach even higher. Then start reaching over gently to the left side, trying to move your upper body and arm in the same direction, as if they were welded together.

DON'TS

❏ **Do not bounce.**

❏ **Do not tense your shoulders or neck.**

❏ **Do not arch your lower back or stick out your stomach.**

❏ When you have reached over to the side as far as you can, move one-sixteenth to one-quarter inch over and back. You should not be making any bouncing or jerking movements, and remember—move in *triple slow motion.*

To reverse sides, or to come out of this exercise, slowly lower your arm and straighten your spine, until you have returned to the original position.

NOTE: If you feel any discomfort in your lower back, or if you have a swayback, you may want to try this exercise with your arms and torso bending slightly forward.

Repetitions
TO EACH SIDE

DAY 1 **25**	DAY 2 **30**	DAY 3 **40**	DAY 4 **50**	5	6	7
8	9	10	11	12	13	14
15	16	17	18	19	20	21
22	23	24	25	26	27	28
29	30					

The Neck Stretch

Relaxation—plain and simple.

THIS EXERCISE: LOOSENS THE NECK AND SHOULDERS • STRETCHES THE SPINE • INCREASES JOINT FLEXIBILITY • RELEASES TENSION IN THE NECK AND BETWEEN THE SHOULDER BLADES

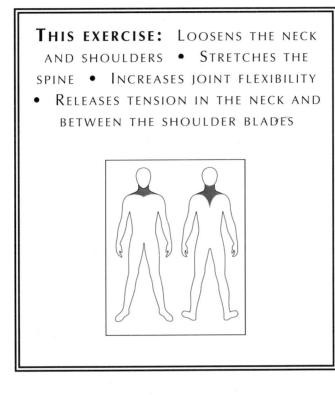

TECHNIQUE

❏ This exercise may be done sitting or standing.

❏ Sit up straight in a chair or stand erect, with your feet forward, a hip-width apart, knees bent. Relax your shoulders and arms.

❏ Stretch your neck up until you feel you can't stretch any higher. Look straight ahead and be conscious that you keep your jaw loose. Feel as if your shoulders were sinking right into the floor and as if a string were running from your head right to the ceiling, stretching your neck even more.

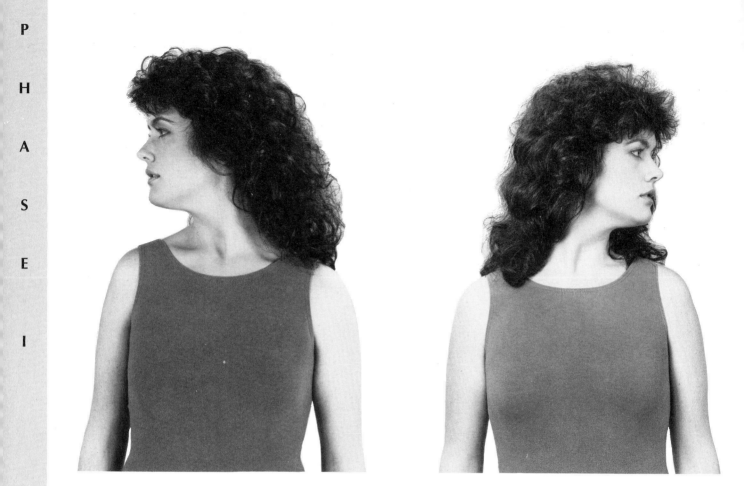

❑ Gently, in *triple slow motion,* turn your head as far as you can to the right until you feel a slight, comfortable stretch. Then, very slowly and in one continuous motion, move it to the left. Try to look over your shoulders, but be sure that you don't rotate them; they should remain facing front. A movement to both sides counts as one repetition.

DON'TS

❑ Do not turn your body or rotate your shoulders.

❑ Do not lock your knees.

❑ Do not tense your neck or shoulders.

❑ Do not stick out your buttocks or your stomach.

Repetitions
TO EACH SIDE

DAY 1	DAY 2	DAY 3	DAY 4	5	6	7
2	3	4	5			
8	9	10	11	12	13	14
15	16	17	18	19	20	21
22	23	24	25	26	27	28
29	30					

The Neck Roll

A way to unlock tension.

THIS EXERCISE: LOOSENS THE NECK AND SHOULDERS • STRETCHES THE SPINE • KEEPS THE NECK AREA FLEXIBLE

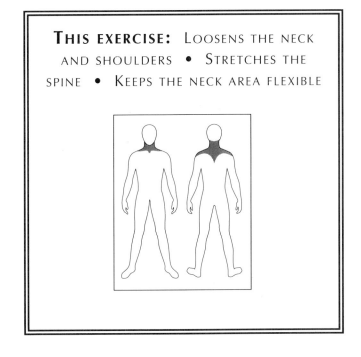

TECHNIQUE

❑ Sit up straight in a chair or stand erect, feet a hip-width apart, knees bent, feet forward. Relax your shoulders—so much so that you feel they are sinking into the floor. Relax your entire body, being careful not to arch your back or stick out your buttocks.

❑ In *triple slow motion*, stretch your neck up. At the same time, lower your chin until it is resting on your chest. Relax your jaw. Relax your shoulders, and try to keep them even and back. Gently, leading with your chin, move your head toward your right shoulder until your nose is even with the middle of your shoulder. Now, look over your shoulder as far as possible, trying to stretch your neck even more. Hold for a slow count of five.

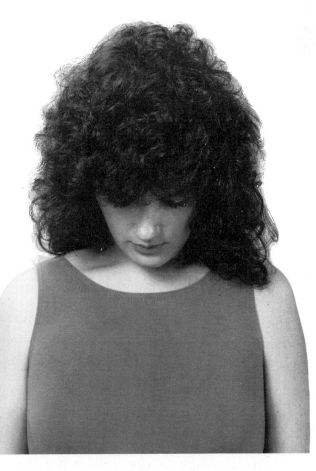

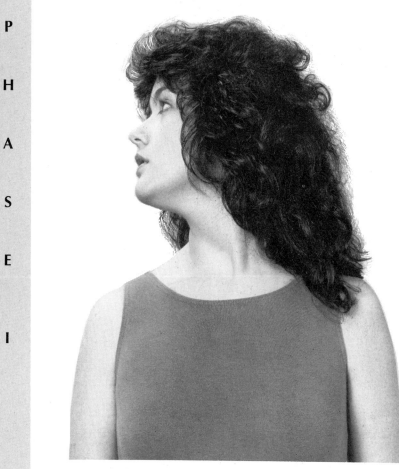

❑ Neck still stretched, slowly bring your chin back down to your chest and move it toward your left shoulder in one continuous slow motion. Look over your left shoulder as far as possible, as on the right side, holding for a slow count of five. Slowly, return your head to the center. This sequence counts as one repetition.

DON'TS

❑ **Do not make any sharp or sudden movements; extreme moves can injure your neck.**

❑ **Do not hunch or tense your shoulders.**

❑ **Do not tense your jaw; it may help to keep your lips slightly apart.**

❑ **Do not lock your knees.**

❑ **Do not stick out your buttocks or stomach.**

Repetitions
TO EACH SIDE

DAY 1	DAY 2	DAY 3	DAY 4	5	6	7
2	3	4	5			
8	9	10	11	12	13	14
15	16	17	18	19	20	21
22	23	24	25	26	27	28
29	30					

THE STOMACH

> **THESE EXERCISES:** STRENGTHEN ALL FOUR GROUPS OF THE ABDOMINAL MUSCLES • LIFT THE BREASTS BY STRENGTHENING THE SUPPORT MUSCLES • REDUCE TENSION IN THE NECK AND UPPER BACK • INCREASE FLEXIBILITY OF THE ENTIRE BACK • REDUCE A DOUBLE CHIN AND MAKE THE NECK APPEAR LONGER • ASSIST IN REGULATING ELIMINATION • HELP TO CONTROL APPETITE (FOR MOST PEOPLE) • HELP LESSEN MONTHLY DISCOMFORT FOR WOMEN

An Important Note

In the beginning, when doing the stomach exercises, you may feel some slight discomfort in the back of the neck area as you round your head and shoulders off the floor. The neck is where many people hold tension, and it is this tension that creates the discomfort. The more tension you hold in your neck, the more you will feel the release of this tension as you keep doing these exercises. Trying to relax as you do the exercises will help, but should you find it too uncomfortable, clasp your hands behind your head and cradle your neck as you perform the movements. The discomfort should not last longer than a few sessions. If soreness in the neck persists, it could be a signal that there is something medically wrong—a call to your doctor is in order.

Remember when you do these exercises that your head, torso, arms, and hands should all move together, as if they were one. Many beginners make the mistake of moving just one body part.

At first you will feel these exercises working just below your chest. The stronger you get, the lower down toward the pubic bone you will feel them. As the upper abdominals begin to pull in, the lower abdomen may appear to protrude. Don't panic (as I did). Unless you have allergies or digestive problems that are causing bloat and need medical attention, your stomach will flatten as the lower abdominals catch up.

The Bent-Knee Reach

You'll never do another sit-up.

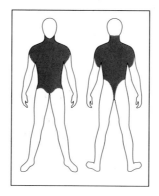

TECHNIQUE

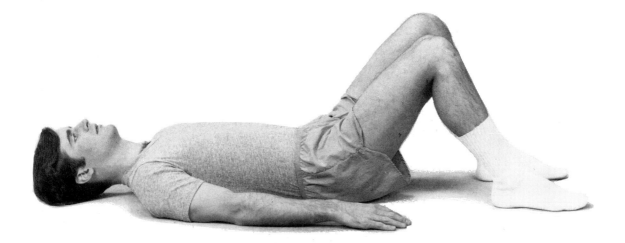

❏ Lie on the floor, your entire body relaxed, knees bent, your feet flat on the floor a hip-width apart, a comfortable distance from your buttocks.

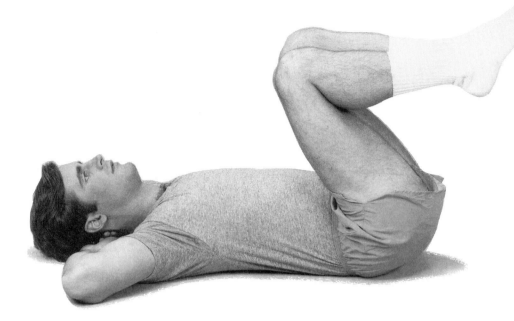

❏ One at a time, bring both knees to your chest. Then, clasp your hands behind your head, just above the neck, and cradle your head in the palms of your hands. Take your elbows out to the sides as much as possible. Do not aim your elbows toward your legs, as this may put too much pressure on the neck.

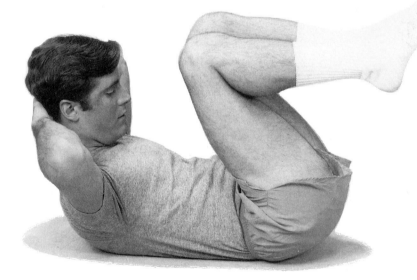

❏ In *triple slow motion*, gently round your head and shoulders off the floor, curling your upper torso and aiming your nose into your chest. When you can't round any more, gently move the upper torso one-sixteenth to one-quarter inch forward and back, within this rounded position. To come out of this position, when repetitions are complete or if you need to take a breather, return your torso to the floor in *triple slow motion*, vertebra by vertebra. Then, one at a time, lower your legs to the floor with knees bent. You can take a breather at any point. To continue, return to the original starting position, making sure your head, shoulders, and upper torso round up gently off the floor.

NOTE: As you progress through Phases I-IV, this exercise will work the entire length of your stomach muscles. You will feel it in different places, with what has best been described as a feeling of "working the muscles in layers, deeper and deeper."

DON'TS

❏ **Do not rock your entire body back and forth.**

❏ **Do not tighten your buttocks.**

❏ **Do not bounce your head or aim it up toward the ceiling.**

❏ **Do not hold in your stomach muscles.**

❏ **Do not hold your breath.**

❏ **Do not lift just your head first.**

Repetitions

DAY 1 25	DAY 2 30	DAY 3 35	DAY 4 40	5	6	7
8	9	10	11	12	13	14
15	16	17	18	19	20	21
22	23	24	25	26	27	28
29	30					

Single-Leg Raises
The fastest way to a flat tummy.

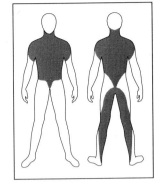

TECHNIQUE

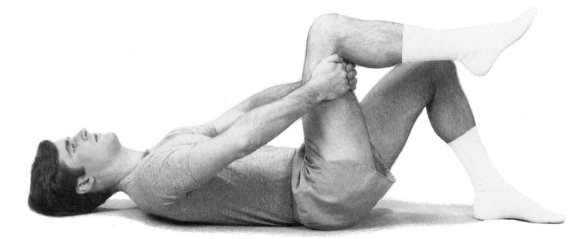

❑ Lie on the floor, with your knees bent, your feet flat on the floor, a hip-width apart, as close to your buttocks as is comfortable.

❑ Raise up your right leg, perpendicular to your body, allowing the knee to remain bent. Be conscious of keeping your leg and toes relaxed.

❑ Keeping your head on the floor, grasp your right leg firmly, with both hands, in back of the thigh, aiming your elbows out to the sides as far as possible. Then point your elbows up as high as possible toward the ceiling.

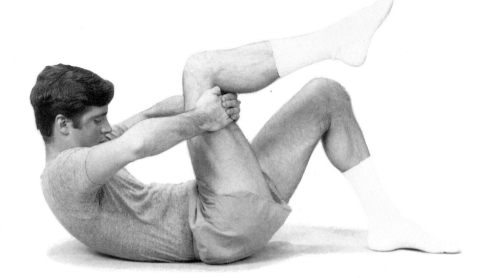

❑ Still grasping your leg firmly, in *triple slow motion*, round your head and upper torso off the floor, trying to aim your nose toward your chest. Slowly, move your upper body one-sixteenth to one-quarter inch forward and back, within the rounded position.

❑ In *triple slow motion*, return your torso to the floor, one vertebra at a time. Then, slowly, lower the raised leg to the starting position. Repeat on the other side. Take breathers when necessary. You will only be able to move a quarter of an inch. This exercise is not about how high you can move, but how rounded you can keep your upper body. Keep your raised leg as perpendicular to the floor as possible.

NOTE: It is very important to learn to relax your entire body when doing this exercise to ensure that you do not try to use your back muscles to compensate for weak stomach muscles.

DON'TS

❑ **Do not tense your toes, knees, or legs.**

❑ **Do not bring the raised leg toward your head, but, rather, round your body toward your leg.**

❑ **Do not rock your body back and forth.**

❑ **Do not jerk up your head.**

❑ **Do not aim your torso toward the ceiling.**

❑ **Do not tense your stomach.**

❑ **Do not tighten your buttocks.**

Repetitions
TO EACH SIDE

DAY 1 25	DAY 2 30	DAY 3 35	DAY 4 40	5	6	7
8	9	10	11	12	13	14
15	16	17	18	19	20	21
22	23	24	25	26	27	28
29	30					

Double-Leg Raises
Flat, flatter, flattest!

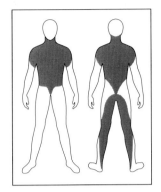

NOTE: To avoid putting any unnecessary pressure on your back, when raising both legs from a lying-down position, you should always remember to bend your knees first and raise them one at a time, before you straighten your legs.

TECHNIQUE

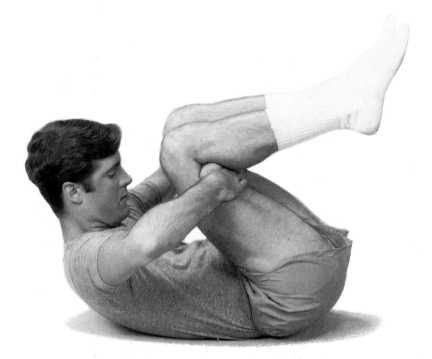

DON'TS

❏ Do not lift up your legs without bending your knees.

❏ Do not tense your legs, knees, or toes.

❏ Do not move only your hands or arms.

❏ Do not jerk your neck.

❏ Do not rock your body back and forth.

❏ Lie on the floor, your entire body relaxed, knees bent, your feet flat on the floor a hip-width apart, a comfortable distance from the buttocks.

❏ One at a time, bring your knees to your chest. Grasp the backs of your thighs, aiming your elbows out to the sides as far as possible. Then point your elbows up as high as possible toward the ceiling.

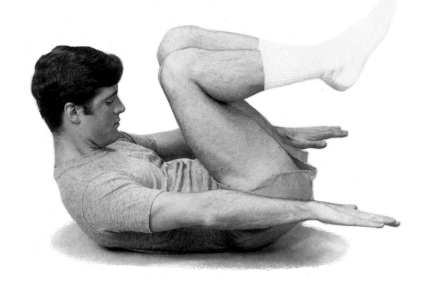

❑ Still holding on to your thighs, in *triple slow motion*, gently round your head and shoulders off the floor, extending your elbows even further out and up, curling your upper torso, and aiming your nose into your chest. When you can't round any more, let go of your thighs and extend your arms out straight by your sides, parallel to and a few inches off the floor, your palms facing downward. Gently, move the upper torso one-sixteenth to one-quarter inch forward and back, within this rounded position. To come out of this position, when repetitions are complete or if you need a breather, return to the floor in *triple slow motion*, vertebra by vertebra. Then, one at a time, lower your feet to the floor, keeping your knees bent. You can take a breather at any point. To continue, return to the original starting position, making sure your head, shoulders, and upper torso round gently off the floor.

Repetitions

DAY 1 25	DAY 2 30	DAY 3 35	DAY 4 40	5	6	7
8	9	10	11	12	13	14
15	16	17	18	19	20	21
22	23	24	25	26	27	28
29	30					

Both Legs Over
To stretch the torso muscles.

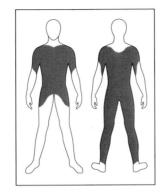

TECHNIQUE

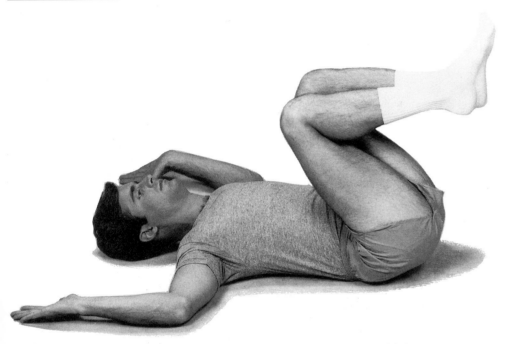

> DON'TS
>
> ❏ **Do not tense or jerk your body; these movements are fluid.**
>
> ❏ **Do not rush through this stretch.**
>
> ❏ **Do not force your legs to the floor.**

❏ Lie on the floor, knees bent, feet on the floor a hip-width apart, a comfortable distance from the buttocks. Your arms are out at shoulder lever, elbows bent up at right angles, the backs of your hands resting on the floor.

❏ In *triple slow motion*, one at a time bring both knees in toward your chest. Take your right leg over to the right side, keeping the leg bent. Let your right leg relax. Then bring over your left leg, resting it on your right leg. Allow gravity to bring your knees as close to the floor as possible. Try to keep your shoulders on the floor. Hold for the count.

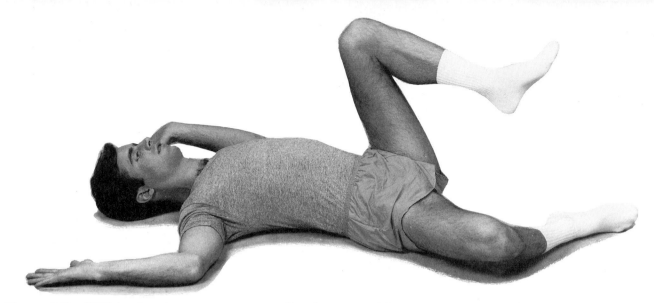

NOTE: Like Will in the picture, you may at first have trouble getting the backs of your hands to rest against the floor. You may also have trouble keeping both elbows on the floor. As you become more stretched, this will get easier.

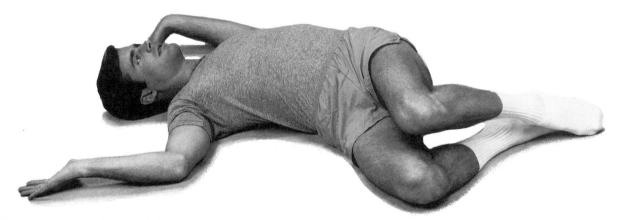

❑ To come out of the position, in *triple slow motion* and one at a time, bend your knees in toward your chest and bring them back to the center. Repeat on the other side.

Hold for a count of . . .
TO EACH SIDE

DAY 1 30	DAY 2 45	DAY 3 60	DAY 4 60	5	6	7
8	9	10	11	12	13	14
15	16	17	18	19	20	21
22	23	24	25	26	27	28
29	30					

The next two exercises are stretches only, and should not involve any muscles other than those of the neck. Now that you've finished your abdominals, this is your chance to let gravity give a further gentle stretch to your neck, hastening even more the release of all that dreadful tension you've been holding for so long—and it's a marvelous opportunity to meditate.

Neck to the Side

To relax the neck.

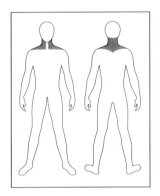

TECHNIQUE

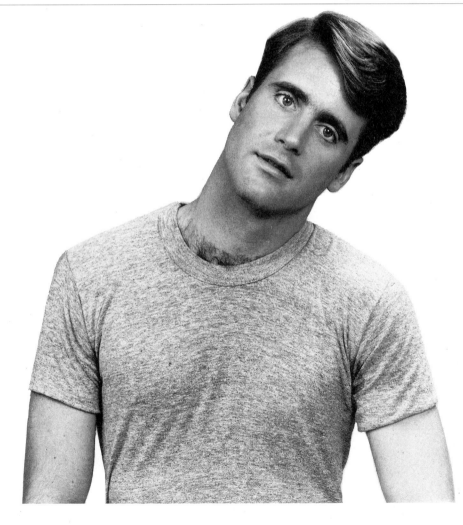

❏ Sit comfortably on the floor. Relax your shoulders.

❏ Keeping your shoulders relaxed and down, in *triple slow motion* allow your head to go over to the right, as though your right ear were going to touch your right shoulder. Hold for a count of ten to fifteen.

❏ Slowly, return your head to an upright position and repeat to the left side. Two movements, one to each side, count as one repetition.

NOTE: When you lower your head to each side, you don't have to do anything but relax and let gravity do the work for you.

DON'TS

❏ **Do not hunch or tense your shoulders.**

❏ **Do not make any jerky movements**

Repetitions
TO EACH SIDE

DAY 1	DAY 2	DAY 3	DAY 4	5	6	7
1	**1**	**1**	**1**			
8	9	10	11	12	13	14
15	16	17	18	19	20	21
22	23	24	25	26	27	28
29	30					

The Three-Quarter Neck Relaxer

To relax the neck.

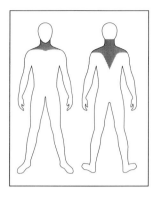

TECHNIQUE

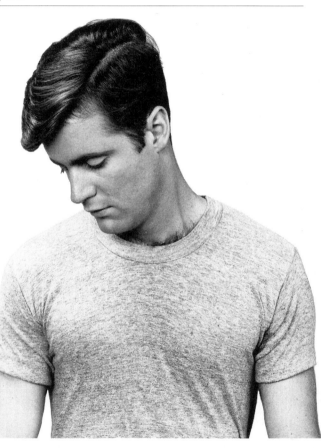

❏ Sit comfortably or stand erect, legs a hip-width apart, knees slightly bent, feet forward. Relax your shoulders.

❏ Try to keep the feeling that your shoulders are melting into the ground as you stretch your neck up. Slowly, turn your head to the right until your chin is halfway between the center and your right shoulder. Allow gravity to lower your head, stretching the back of your neck. Feel as if you were trying to touch your chin to your collarbone. Hold for a count of ten to fifteen.

❏ In *triple slow motion*, raise your head and slowly return to the original position. Gently, turn your head to the left and repeat the movement, holding for a count of ten to fifteen. Slowly, return to the center.

Repetitions
TO EACH SIDE

DAY 1	DAY 2	DAY 3	DAY 4	5	6	7
1	**1**	**1**	**1**			
8	9	10	11	12	13	14
15	16	17	18	19	20	21
22	23	24	25	26	27	28
29	30					

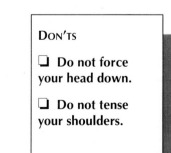

DON'TS

❏ **Do not force your head down.**

❏ **Do not tense your shoulders.**

LEGS AND INNER THIGHS

NOTE: If you have knee problems, do this exercise and the next very gently and slowly. They should not aggravate any existing problems. In fact, many students with knee problems due to injuries, arthritis, or even surgery have reported that these exercises improved their conditions tremendously. Just be cautious and use your judgment. You'll find that practising these exercises can actually help decrease the likelihood of future injuries in any activity by strengthening your leg muscles. Since these muscles are the same ones that assist the back muscles in everyday activities, the extra bonus is that you'll be less likely to have any problems running, walking, or standing.

Bend and Curl

The way to leaner, longer-looking legs.

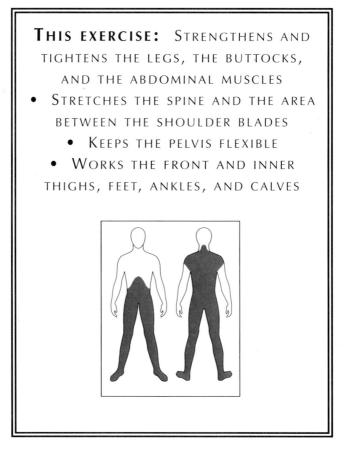

THIS EXERCISE: STRENGTHENS AND TIGHTENS THE LEGS, THE BUTTOCKS, AND THE ABDOMINAL MUSCLES
• STRETCHES THE SPINE AND THE AREA BETWEEN THE SHOULDER BLADES
• KEEPS THE PELVIS FLEXIBLE
• WORKS THE FRONT AND INNER THIGHS, FEET, ANKLES, AND CALVES

❏ Face a "barre." You may use the top of a table, counter, desk, back of the sofa, heavy chair, or anything that can support your weight, but whatever you use should not be lower than the middle of your thighs. Hold on to the "barre" with straight, yet relaxed arms. You should be about twelve to eighteen inches away from your "barre." Heels are a comfortable distance apart, knees bent, feet turned out. Relax your body totally.

DON'TS

❏ **Do not stick out your buttocks or stomach.**

❏ **Do not allow your buttocks to drop lower than your knees.**

❏ **Do not tense your shoulders.**

❏ Keeping your spine as straight as possible, shoulders back, bend your knees to lower your body one inch toward the floor. Then tighten your buttocks and curl up your pelvis in *triple slow motion*. With a little extra effort, you can curl up your pelvis even more than you think. Hold for a count of five, then slowly release your pelvis.

❏ Lower your body one inch more. Curl up your pelvis and hold for a count of five, then slowly release it. Reverse the process: come back up one inch, curl your pelvis, and hold for another five counts, release, come up one inch more, curl pelvis, hold five, release. This entire sequence is one repetition.

NOTE: At first you will not realize how much your pelvis can curl up with a beautiful, smooth flow. The more you relax your body, the easier this will be and the faster you will progress.

Repetitions

DAY 1	DAY 2	DAY 3	DAY 4	5	6	7
2	**2**	**3**	**3**			
8	9	10	11	12	13	14
15	16	17	18	19	20	21
22	23	24	25	26	27	28
29	30					

Plié and Balance

A great toner for legs.

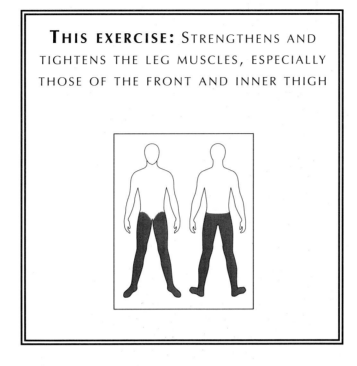

THIS EXERCISE: STRENGTHENS AND TIGHTENS THE LEG MUSCLES, ESPECIALLY THOSE OF THE FRONT AND INNER THIGH

TECHNIQUE

❏ Face the "barre," standing about twelve to eighteen inches away from it, and hold it with straight, yet relaxed arms. Your legs are relaxed, knees bent, feet flat on the floor, slightly turned out, a comfortable distance apart.

In *triple slow motion*, gently bend your knees to lower your body as far as you can without having to lift your heels off the floor. Trying to keep your body straight, your spine as erect as possible, return to the original position and repeat. Rather than holding the lowered position, try to make this one continuous up-and-down motion. But, remember—do it in *triple slow motion*.

NOTE: *If your leg muscles are weak, at first you may feel as if you are clinging to the "barre" with every muscle in your body. Even your teeth will feel as if they are trying to hold you up! As you gain strength in your legs, you will automatically be able to stand more erect and you will find yourself an arm's length away from the "barre," with your hands only touching it lightly for balance.*

DON'TS

❑ **Do not stick out your buttocks or your stomach.**

❑ **Do not tense your shoulders.**

Repetitions

DAY 1	DAY 2	DAY 3	DAY 4	5	6	7
5	**7**	**9**	**10**			
8	9	10	11	12	13	14
15	16	17	18	19	20	21
22	23	24	25	26	27	28
29	30					

Up and Over

If this leg stretch aggravates your sciatica or other lower-back problems, skip to the following exercise, which provides an alternate stretch, and do twice as many repetitions as are called for.

THIS EXERCISE: STRETCHES THE NECK, SPINE, BETWEEN THE SHOULDER BLADES, THE BUTTOCKS, THE INNER THIGHS, THE HAMSTRING MUSCLES, AND THE CALVES

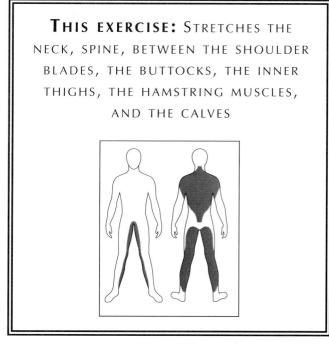

NOTE: Find out what your limitations are by gently trying different positions and heights before you begin.

TECHNIQUE

❑ For this exercise, whatever you are using as a "barre" should be even with or lower than your knee, such as a low chair or sofa. Face the "barre" and gently place your right heel on it, keeping the standing foot facing forward with the knee bent as much as possible. (You may have to turn the foot out slightly for balance.) Keep the raised right leg bent, and relax the standing leg as well. Place your hands, one in front of the other, on your right thigh. Hold your elbows out to the sides to stretch between your shoulder blades.

DON'TS

❑ **Do not lock either of your knees.**

❑ **Do not rest your hands on your knees.**

❑ **Do not make jerking movements with your neck or torso.**

❑ **Do not tense your neck or shoulders.**

❏ In *triple slow motion*, your hands still resting on your thighs, move your torso toward your knee until you feel a stretch, then hold until you feel the muscles relax and you can stretch a little further. Hold, then gently move the torso one-sixteenth to one-quarter inch toward the knee and back. If you already feel a strong stretch, simply hold the position for the count. Keep your entire body relaxed, especially your neck and knees. To come out of this stretch, raise your torso, and gently, in *triple slow motion*, lift the leg off the "barre" and return it to the floor. Repeat with your left leg.

NOTE: *If you want more of a stretch than you are able to get in this position, gently scoot the standing leg further back from the "barre" and try to straighten the raised leg as much as possible. If you find that the "barre" cuts into your ankle uncomfortably, cushion it with a thick cloth or towel.*

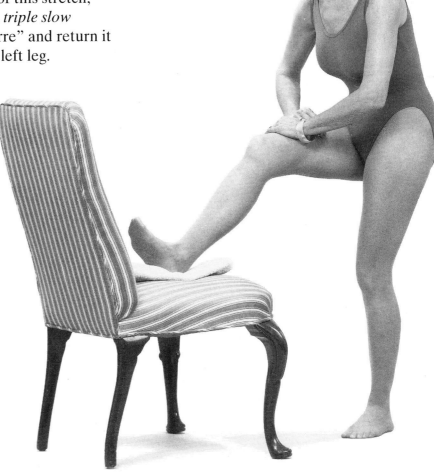

Repetitions
TO EACH SIDE

DAY 1 15	DAY 2 20	DAY 3 25	DAY 4 25	5	6	7
8	9	10	11	12	13	14
15	16	17	18	19	20	21
22	23	24	25	26	27	28
29	30					

Hamstring Stretch

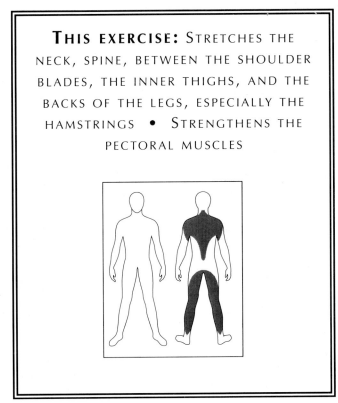

THIS EXERCISE: STRETCHES THE NECK, SPINE, BETWEEN THE SHOULDER BLADES, THE INNER THIGHS, AND THE BACKS OF THE LEGS, ESPECIALLY THE HAMSTRINGS • STRENGTHENS THE PECTORAL MUSCLES

TECHNIQUE

❏ Lie on your back, your entire body relaxed, knees bent, your feet flat on the floor a hip-width apart, a comfortable distance from your buttocks. Your arms are resting at your sides.

DON'TS

❏ Do not bounce.

❏ Do not force the raised leg forward by pulling it.

❏ Do not force the raised leg to straighten.

❏ Do not tense your neck.

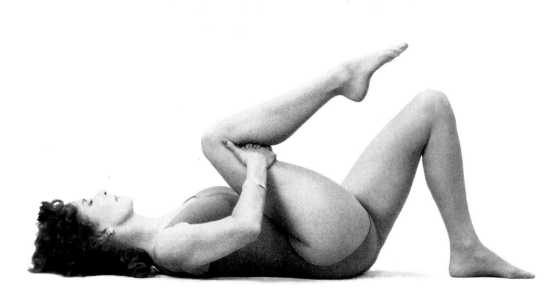

❏ Bend your right knee and, holding the back of your right thigh below the knee with both hands, elbows out to the side, bring your leg as close as possible toward your chin. Keeping your head on the floor, slowly straighten your leg as much as you can, aiming it upward without forcing it. Straighten it only as much as is comfortable.

❏ Hold for a count of ten and then gently move your right leg toward you and back one-sixteenth to one-quarter inch. It is very important that these delicate movements do not even resemble a bounce. If you really feel the stretch in your leg, simply hold for the count. To come out of this position, release your arms, and in *triple slow motion* return the raised leg to the starting position. Repeat to the left side.

NOTE: The hamstring muscle is usually the tightest muscle in the body. In fact, a large percentage of the population have extremely tight hamstrings. So be patient. It may take longer than thirty days to stretch this muscle completely. Just be aware that your muscles are stretching every time you do this exercise. And every little bit counts! As you become more flexible day by day, try to gradually increase the length of the count you hold the stretch from ten to thirty seconds, before you begin the repetitions.

Repetitions
TO EACH SIDE

DAY 1 15	DAY 2 20	DAY 3 25	DAY 4 30	5	6	7
8	9	10	11	12	13	14
15	16	17	18	19	20	21
22	23	24	25	26	27	28
29	30					

The Standing Stretch

For the top of the thighs.

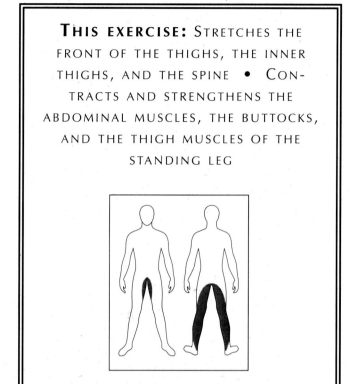

THIS EXERCISE: STRETCHES THE FRONT OF THE THIGHS, THE INNER THIGHS, AND THE SPINE • CONTRACTS AND STRENGTHENS THE ABDOMINAL MUSCLES, THE BUTTOCKS, AND THE THIGH MUSCLES OF THE STANDING LEG

❑ Face the "barre" or the wall, resting your left hand on it. Stand straight, your feet a hip-width apart, your body relaxed. Bend your right knee and lift your right foot behind you so that you can hold it loosely in your right hand. It should not touch your right buttock. Your right foot should now be aimed upward. Bend the standing leg very slightly. Hold for the count.

❑ Slowly, release and lower your right foot. Repeat on the other side.

DON'TS

❑ Do not let the foot of the bent leg touch your buttocks.

❑ Do not arch your back or stick out your stomach.

❑ Do not lock your elbows or the knee of the standing leg.

Hold for a count of . . .
TO EACH SIDE

DAY 1 10	DAY 2 15	DAY 3 20	DAY 4 30	5	6	7
8	9	10	11	12	13	14
15	16	17	18	19	20	21
22	23	24	25	26	27	28
29	30					

The Inner-Thigh Tightener

As we get older, our inner thighs start to look like plastic bags filled with Jell-O. This exercise will give you lethal inner thighs.

THIS EXERCISE: TIGHTENS THE INNER THIGHS • STRETCHES THE SPINE • STRENGTHENS THE STOMACH, BUTTOCKS, PSOAS, CALVES, AND FEET

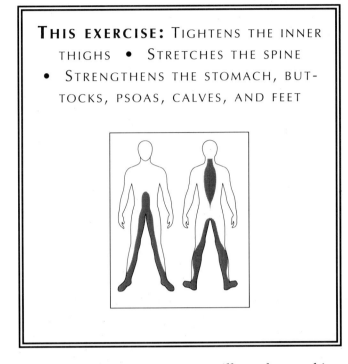

NOTE: *For this exercise, you will need something sturdy that you can squeeze with your legs. You can use a desk, a coffee or tea table, a chair—or even something like a filing cabinet. Its width is not critical, as long as you are comfortable. Just make sure that it's not fragile. You may be surprised at how strong your inner thighs will become as you do this powerful contraction.*

TECHNIQUE

❏ Sit on the floor, in front of whatever you will be squeezing, your legs straight on the floor. Bend your knees and wrap the arches of your feet around the sides of the object. Next, round your upper back, allowing your shoulders to collapse and slouch slightly. Keep your arms relaxed, and rest your palms on the floor at your sides. If you try to sit up too fast too soon, you will be forcing your lower back to do much of the work.

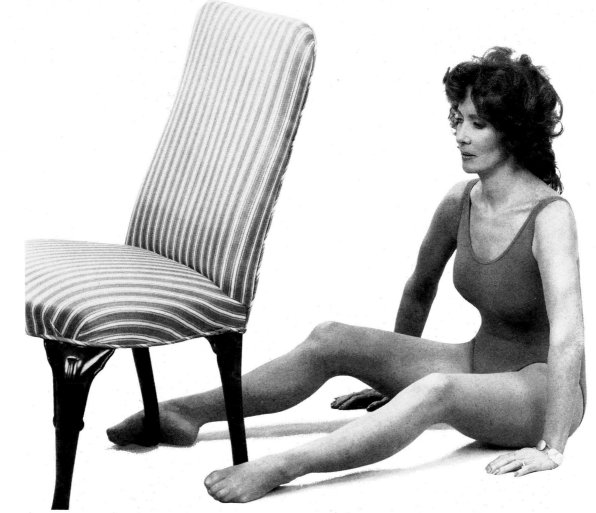

❏ Keeping your knees bent, apply pressure with your feet and try to squeeze them together as hard as you can. Squeeze for the count, if you can, then release. You will see much better results if you squeeze continuously, instead of holding and relaxing.

NOTE: *At first you may feel this exercise mostly in the calves and inside of the knees. As you progress, you'll feel it working the inner thighs.*

DON'TS

❏ **Do not squeeze and release; hold steadily for the count.**

❏ **Do not tense your shoulders.**

Hold for a count of . . .

DAY 1 25	DAY 2 25	DAY 3 25	DAY 4 25	5	6	7
8	9	10	11	12	13	14
15	16	17	18	19	20	21
22	23	24	25	26	27	28
29	30					

BUTTOCKS, HIPS, AND OUTER THIGHS

PLEASE NOTE: This series of exercises may appear complicated at first. Please be sure to read through the text to get an understanding of what you must do before attempting them. The benefits will be well worth it. Don't worry about doing these exercises at exactly the level shown in the photographs. Do them at your own level, which is perfect for you. As your muscles strengthen, your form will improve. Don't be discouraged if you feel that you are starting over again at each new phase. You'll be working the muscles deeper and deeper, and in no time at all each phase will be a breeze.

> **THE NEXT TWO EXERCISES:** SCULPT THE BUTTOCKS, GIVING THEM A "PRECIOUS PEACH" (INSTEAD OF A "SAGGING PEAR") SHAPE • GET RID OF THE "JIGGLE" • REDUCE SADDLEBAGS, AND EVENTUALLY MAKE THEM DISAPPEAR • STRENGTHEN THE ARM MUSCLES

Bringing Up the Rear

You'll feel this one working!

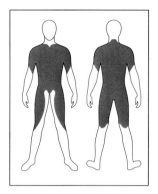

TECHNIQUE

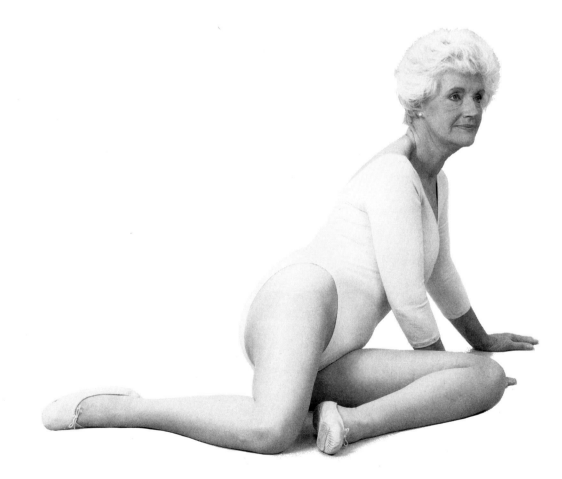

❑ Sit on your left buttock, with your left knee bent, resting comfortably on the floor in front of you, your heel away from your body. Your right leg is out to the side, your right knee bent and even with your left arch. Your right foot is to the back. Lean your torso to the left and then straighten your back (so that you aren't tempted to arch it). Rest your hands on the floor, anywhere between your knee and hip. Your elbows should be slightly bent.

❑ Lift your right leg so that your knee is several inches off the floor. Gently, in *triple slow motion*, move your right knee one-sixteenth to one-quarter inch back and return. After you have completed your repetitions, slowly lower it to the floor.

❑ Reverse and repeat the exercise to the other side.

NOTE: This exercise is based on a ballet position called an "attitude." I have modified it so that it works the buttock muscles even more deeply. If you are having trouble raising your leg, move your hands further away from your body and try leaning over to the side more. This will make it easier to lift your leg.

DON'TS

❑ Do not stick out your buttocks.

❑ Do not tense any part of your body, especially your shoulders.

❑ Do not push out your stomach.

❑ Do not arch your back.

Repetitions
TO EACH SIDE

DAY 1	DAY 2	DAY 3	DAY 4	5	6	7
15	**20**	**25**	**25**			
8	9	10	11	12	13	14
15	16	17	18	19	20	21
22	23	24	25	26	27	28
29	30					

Out to the Side

For a great back view!

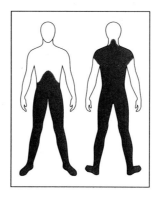

TECHNIQUE

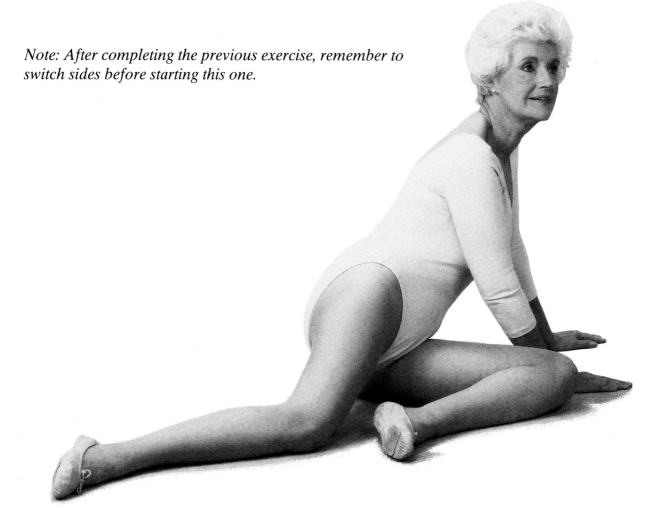

Note: After completing the previous exercise, remember to switch sides before starting this one.

❑ Sit on the left buttock, with your left leg resting comfortably on the floor in front of you, your knee bent and your heel away from your body. Your right leg is resting out to the side on the floor, slightly in front of your hip, knee bent, so that your right knee is even with your left arch. Lean to your left side and rest your hands on the floor, anywhere between your knee and hip. Your elbows should be slightly bent.

❏ Lift your right leg as much as you can, but no more than eight inches off the floor. Gently, move your entire leg up and down one-sixteenth to one-quarter inch. Alternate sides, working up to the required number of repetitions by breaking it up into sets if you have to.

NOTE: Lean to the side as far as necessary to get your legs into the correct position.

DON'TS

❏ Do not stick out your stomach.

❏ Do not arch your back.

❏ Do not tense your neck or shoulders.

Repetitions TO EACH SIDE						
DAY 1 **15**	DAY 2 **20**	DAY 3 **25**	DAY 4 **25**	5	6	7
8	9	10	11	12	13	14
15	16	17	18	19	20	21
22	23	24	25	26	27	28
29	30					

Pelvic Circles

This exercise and the next are based on a series I learned when studying belly dancing. Everyone loves to show off the flexibility they get from this one in particular. Try it, and you'll see that Elvis had the right idea.

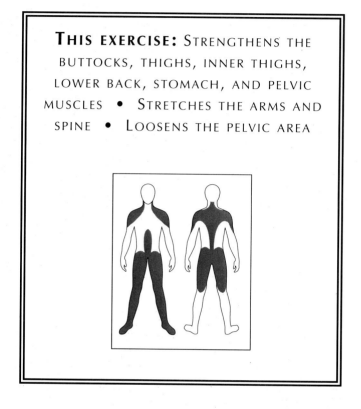

THIS EXERCISE: STRENGTHENS THE BUTTOCKS, THIGHS, INNER THIGHS, LOWER BACK, STOMACH, AND PELVIC MUSCLES • STRETCHES THE ARMS AND SPINE • LOOSENS THE PELVIC AREA

NOTE: Almost everyone finds this exercise difficult to do at first. This is because pelvic circles involve most of the muscle groups in your body. You've probably never even used some of them separately, never mind asking them to join together to do something they've never done before! So don't judge yourself; just do the best you can. Every time you do this exercise, you will be building strength in all these different muscles, and you will start to appreciate the benefits of this beautiful, flowing, seductive movement. Loosening the pelvic area is important. The legs and torso are influenced by it tremendously, and if this area is tight, you won't have the flexibility that everyone is entitled to. This exercise can help you regain the wonderful youthful suppleness and sense of freedom you had as a child.

❑ Knees a hip-width apart, kneel on a pillow or something large enough to cushion your legs from knee to foot. Place your hands on your hips and lower your torso three inches.

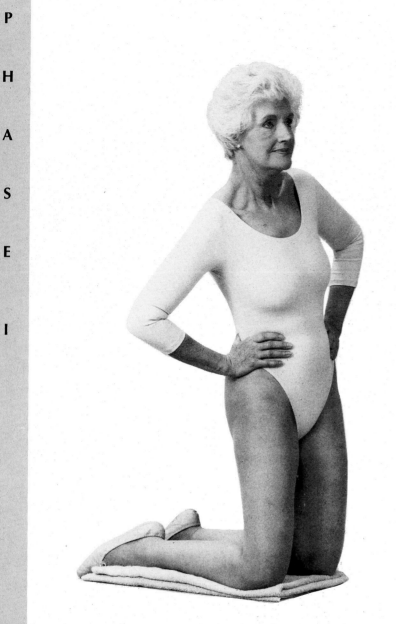

DON'TS

❏ **Do not arch your back.**

❏ **Do not stick out your stomach.**

❏ **Do not try to do too much too fast.**

❏ In *triple slow motion*, gently begin to move your hips (not your torso) as far as you can to the right. Then, slowly, rotate your pelvis to the front. Try to aim your pelvis up toward your navel, then slowly begin to rotate your hips as far as you can to the left side. Then aim your buttocks to your back, being careful not to arch your lower back, but rather trying to stretch to your back so that you feel the stretch in the lower part of your spine. This completes one movement. Working at your own pace, complete the repetitions to this side, circling to the right, front, left, and back. Then take a breather if you feel you need it before reversing direction.

Repetitions
IN EACH DIRECTION

DAY 1 2	DAY 2 2	DAY 3 2	DAY 4 2	5	6	7
8	9	10	11	12	13	14
15	16	17	18	19	20	21
22	23	24	25	26	27	28
29	30					

The Pelvic Dip

Graceful, flowing . . . beautifying.

THIS EXERCISE: STRENGTHENS THE
LEG MUSCLES, ESPECIALLY THE FRONT-
AND INNER-THIGH MUSCLES, THE
STOMACH, BUTTOCKS, AND CALVES
• STRETCHES THE SPINE

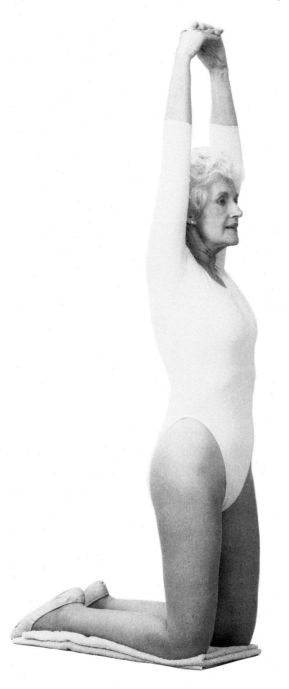

DON'TS

❏ **Do not arch your back.**

❏ **Do not jerk up your pelvis.**

❏ Knees a hip-width apart, kneel on a pillow or something large enough to cushion your legs from knee to foot. Try to bring your arms straight up over your head, clasp your hands, and try to stretch your upper body, including your neck, as if you were trying to make your torso longer. Do this to the point where you can feel your lower back stretching.

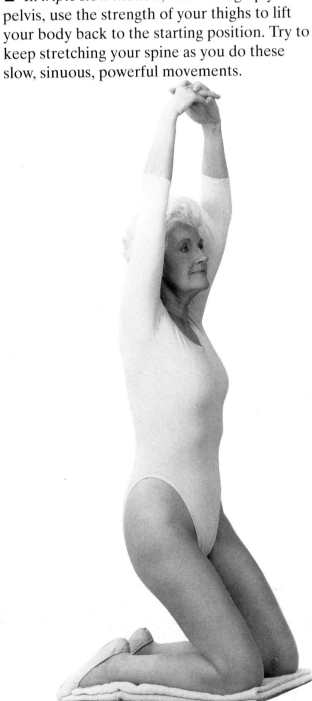

❑ Continue to stretch as you slowly lower your buttocks about four inches, then tighten your buttock muscles and slowly curl up your pelvis. Hold this position for a count of three. Your arms will move forward when you tip the pelvis.

❑ In *triple slow motion*, still curling up your pelvis, use the strength of your thighs to lift your body back to the starting position. Try to keep stretching your spine as you do these slow, sinuous, powerful movements.

Repetitions

DAY 1	DAY 2	DAY 3	DAY 4	5	6	7
2	2	2	2			
8	9	10	11	12	13	14
15	16	17	18	19	20	21
22	23	24	25	26	27	28
29	30					

The Front-Thigh Stretch

For tight, slim, beautiful thighs.

THIS EXERCISE: STRETCHES THE
NECK, PECTORAL MUSCLES, SPINE, AND
THIGHS • STRENGTHENS THE BUT-
TOCKS, INNER THIGHS, AND STOMACH

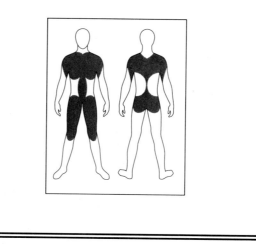

TECHNIQUE

❑ Kneel on a pillow or something large enough
to cushion your legs from knee to toe. Place your
knees together and sit back on your heels. Support yourself by making fists with your hands
and place them on the floor at your sides, so that
they are even with your toes. Still on your heels,
tighten your buttocks and curl up your pelvis.
Hold this position for the count.

❏ Return to the original position by releasing your buttocks and, still sitting on your heels, using your fists to "walk" yourself to an upright position. Relax.

NOTE: The more you can curl up your pelvis, the more you will stretch your thigh muscles. This stretch complements the pelvic exercises you have been doing, and will prevent the development of bulky muscles. If this stretch is too difficult, do the standing hamstring stretch on page 63 until you are ready to tackle this one.

page 63

DON'TS

❏ Do not arch your back or stick out your stomach.

❏ Do not tense your body.

❏ Do not hunch your shoulders.

Hold for a count of . . .

DAY 1 10	DAY 2 10	DAY 3 15	DAY 4 15	5	6	7
8	9	10	11	12	13	14
15	16	17	18	19	20	21
22	23	24	25	26	27	28
29	30					

The Crossover

To release those muscles you've been working so hard.

THIS EXERCISE: STRETCHES THE ENTIRE BACK, SPINE, BETWEEN THE SHOULDER BLADES, PECTORALS, BUTTOCKS, HIPS, AND OUTER THIGHS

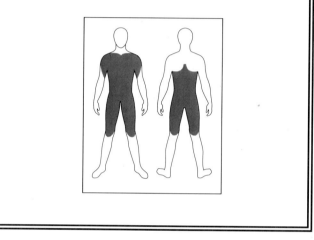

TECHNIQUE

❑ Lie on the floor, knees bent, feet flat on the floor a hip-width apart. Extend your arms out at shoulder level, elbows bent up at right angles, so that the backs of your hands rest on the floor.

❑ Bring your right knee toward your chest. Slide your left foot forward so that your leg is fully extended on the floor. Keeping your right leg bent, bring it over to your left as far as you can, so that your right foot is resting on your left leg, anywhere that is comfortable except directly on top of the kneecap. Allow gravity to lower your right knee as close to the floor as possible, keeping your right leg relaxed. Try to keep your shoulders and elbows on the floor. Hold for the count.

❑ To come out of this position, in *triple slow motion* return your bent right knee to your chest and then slowly lower your right foot to the floor, keeping the knee bent. Bring your left leg to your chest and repeat on the other side.

NOTE: If your muscles are stretched enough, after a count of ten, still resting your foot on the extended leg, move the bent knee toward the floor and back no more than one-sixteenth of an inch in triple slow motion fifteen times.

Like Lucy in the picture, you may have trouble at first getting the backs of your hands to lie flat against the floor.

Hold for a count of . . .
TO EACH SIDE

DAY 1	DAY 2	DAY 3	DAY 4	5	6	7
25	**25**	**25**	**25**			
8	9	10	11	12	13	14
15	16	17	18	19	20	21
22	23	24	25	26	27	28
29	30					

DON'TS

❑ Do not lift your shoulders off the floor.

❑ Do not bring your elbows off the floor.

❑ Do not turn your head to either side.

❑ Do not jerk your bent knee.

❑ Do not force the stretch.

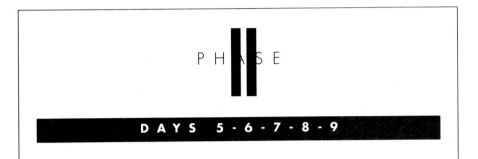

PH A S E

II

By now, any initial soreness should have disappeared, as your body starts to understand the way your muscles are working and why.

As you move into this next phase, you must concentrate very hard. Now that you are more familiar with the exercises, you will also become more conscious of the need to relax. With every motion that you make, pretend that your body is like butter melting in the sun. You will see that you can relax, and you will notice right away when you are not relaxed. You are starting to be in control, so you must make the choice and take the responsibility. By constantly reminding yourself, you will relax more and more, and you will consequently be able to complete more repetitions without taking as many breathers.

The one area where this may not be true is the stomach. As you work the stomach muscles more deeply, day by day, you may find that you can't do as many repetitions as you did the day before. This is natural. Take breathers, keep going, and gradually you will work up to your previous level—and surpass it.

By the end of this phase, you'll start to feel your muscles working deeply, tightening and pulling up. Keep going, and very soon you'll be able to see the difference in the mirror.

WARM-UPS

The Underarm Tightener

TECHNIQUE

❑ Repeat the exercise as in Phase I, trying to keep your head and body as erect as possible. Hold your arms up as high as you can. You may find that, sitting straight, you cannot raise your arms as high as you did in Phase I. If your chair has a high back, you'll need to straddle it backward, as pictured, to keep it from getting in your way.

NOTE: The more you rotate your arms, the more your palms face upward, and the higher your arms are held, the more you will feel this exercise and the faster it will work!

Don'ts

❏ Do not jerk your arms back and forth.

❏ Do not arch your back or stick out your stomach.

❏ Do not lock your elbows.

❏ Do not tense your shoulders.

Repetitions

1	2	3	4	DAY 5 **30**	DAY 6 **40**	DAY 7 **50**
DAY 8 **60**	DAY 9 **75**	10	11	12	13	14
15	16	17	18	19	20	21
22	23	24	25	26	27	28
29	30					

The Waist Away

TECHNIQUE

❏ Stand next to a "barre" (chair back, table, or dresser, for example) with feet a hip-width apart, facing forward, knees bent and relaxed. Rest your left hand or arm on the "barre." Keeping your spine erect, slowly stretch your right arm upward, palm facing inward. Try to keep your arm by your ear. Still stretching upward, tighten your buttocks and curl up your pelvis. Then start reaching over to the left side. Complete the exercise as in Phase I, bending both knees deeply as you come out of the position. Work both sides.

NOTE: At first you may have to do this exercise bent slightly forward, and you may not be able to keep the raised arm straight or by your ear. As you get stronger, your torso will be able to stretch over to the side more, and instead of just feeling the stretch in your waist, you will feel it from your hip to your hand!

DON'TS

❏ Do not bounce.

❏ Do not tense your shoulders or neck.

❏ Do not arch your lower back or stick out your stomach.

❏ Do not lock your knees.

Repetitions
TO EACH SIDE

1	2	3	4	DAY 5 30	DAY 6 40	DAY 7 50
DAY 8 60	DAY 9 75	10	11	12	13	14
15	16	17	18	19	20	21
22	23	24	25	26	27	28
29	30					

The Neck Stretch

TECHNIQUE

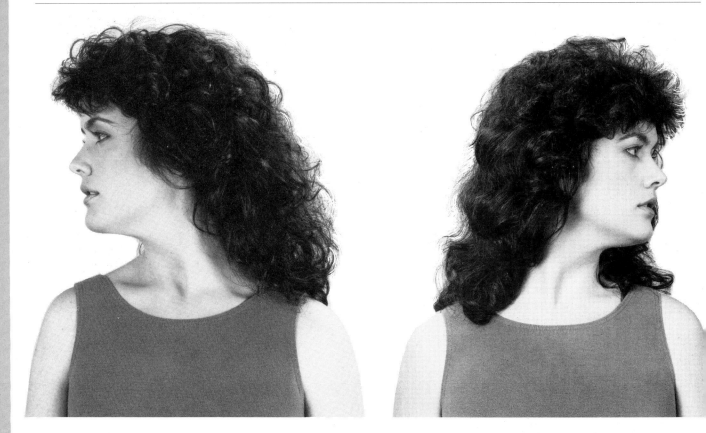

❏ Repeat as in Phase I. If you have been doing this exercise sitting down, now do it standing, with knees bent.

NOTE: As your body learns to relax, you will be able to perform these movements more smoothly.

Repetitions
TO EACH SIDE

1	2	3	4	DAY 5 5	DAY 6 5	DAY 7 5
DAY 8 5	DAY 9 5	10	11	12	13	14
15	16	17	18	19	20	21
22	23	24	25	26	27	28
29	30					

DON'TS

❏ Do not turn your body or rotate your shoulders.

❏ Do not lock your knees.

❏ Do not tense your neck or shoulders.

❏ Do not stick out your buttocks or stomach.

The Neck Roll

TECHNIQUE

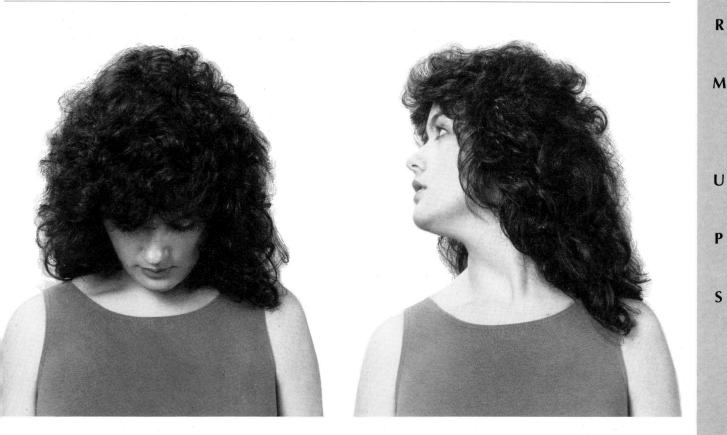

❏ Repeat as in Phase I. If you have been doing this exercise sitting down, now do it standing, with knees bent. As your muscles relax and become stretched, you will find that you can stretch further without tensing your shoulders.

Repetitions
TO EACH SIDE

1	2	3	4	DAY 5 5	DAY 6 5	DAY 7 5
DAY 8 5	DAY 9 5	10	11	12	13	14
15	16	17	18	19	20	21
22	23	24	25	26	27	28
29	30					

DON'TS

❏ **Do not make any sharp or sudden movements.**

❏ **Do not hunch or tense your shoulders.**

❏ **Do not tense your jaw.**

❏ **Do not lock your knees.**

❏ **Do not stick out your stomach or arch your back.**

THE STOMACH

The Bent-Knee Reach

TECHNIQUE

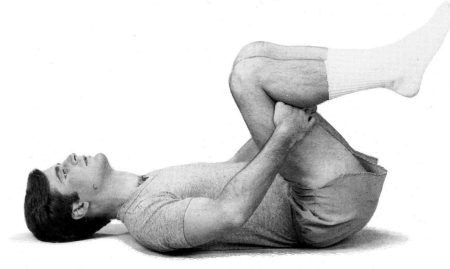

❏ Repeat as in Phase I, but this time, instead of clasping your hands behind your head, grasp the back of your thighs. Still holding on to your thighs, in *triple slow motion* gently round your head and shoulders off the floor, curling your upper torso until your nose is aiming into your chest. Complete the exercise as in Phase I.

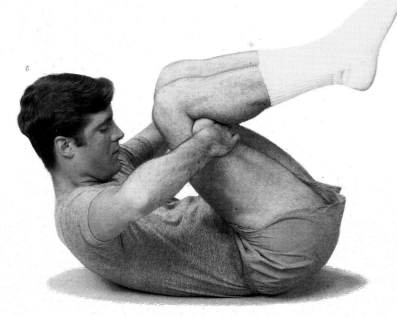

DON'TS

❏ Do not rock your entire body back and forth.

❏ Do not tighten your buttocks.

❏ Do not bounce your head or aim it toward the ceiling.

❏ Do not hold in your stomach muscles.

❏ Do not hold your breath.

❏ Do not lift just your head first.

Repetitions

1	2	3	4	DAY 5 30	DAY 6 40	DAY 7 50
DAY 8 60	DAY 9 70	10	11	12	13	14
15	16	17	18	19	20	21
22	23	24	25	26	27	28
29	30					

Single Leg Raises

TECHNIQUE

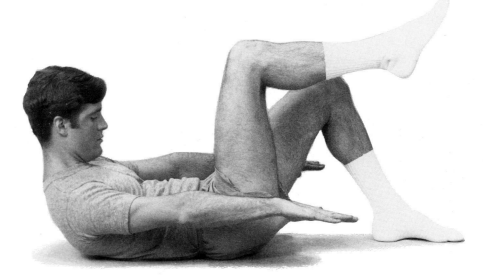

❏ Repeat as in Phase I, this time letting go of your leg and placing your arms straight out alongside your legs, parallel to the floor. Then move your upper body one-sixteenth to one-quarter inch forward and back. Work both sides.

NOTE: Should you feel this exercise in your lower back, lower your torso toward the floor one sixteenth of an inch while continuing the exercise. If you still feel it, try another sixteenth of an inch, and keep on lowering your torso in this manner until you no longer feel it in your back.

DON'TS

❏ Do not tense your toes, knees, or legs.

❏ Do not bring your raised leg toward your head, but rather round your body toward your leg.

❏ Do not rock your body back and forth.

❏ Do not jerk up your head.

❏ Do not aim your torso toward the ceiling.

❏ Do not tense your stomach.

❏ Do not forcibly tighten your buttocks.

❏ Do not move your hands or arms.

Repetitions
TO EACH SIDE

1	2	3	4	DAY 5 40	DAY 6 40	DAY 7 50
DAY 8 60	DAY 9 70	10	11	12	13	14
15	16	17	18	19	20	21
22	23	24	25	26	27	28
29	30					

Double-Leg Raises

TECHNIQUE

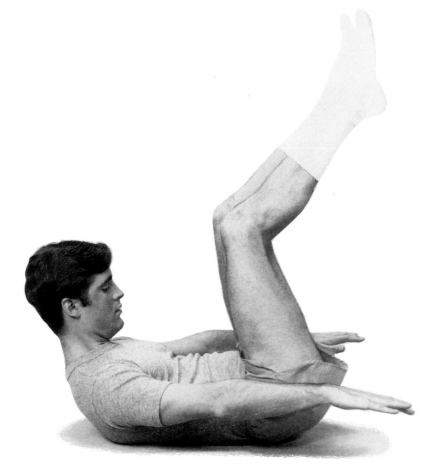

❏ Repeat as in Phase I, but this time, after bending your knees to your chest, raise your legs up, straightening them as much as you can. *Do not force.* After you have rounded up, release your arms so that they are straight out at your sides, a few inches off the floor, palms facing downward. Complete as in Phase I.

NOTE: In the exercises where one or both legs are raised, you will have the added advantage of stretching your hamstring muscle as you work on your stomach. On many people, this muscle is very tight, so remember not to force the leg to straighten. Be patient. Your muscle knows best, and it will stretch on its own timetable, when it's ready to and not before.

Repetitions

1	2	3	4	DAY 5 30	DAY 6 40	DAY 7 50
DAY 8 60	DAY 9 70	10	11	12	13	14
15	16	17	18	19	20	21
22	23	24	25	26	27	28
29	30					

Both Legs Over

TECHNIQUE

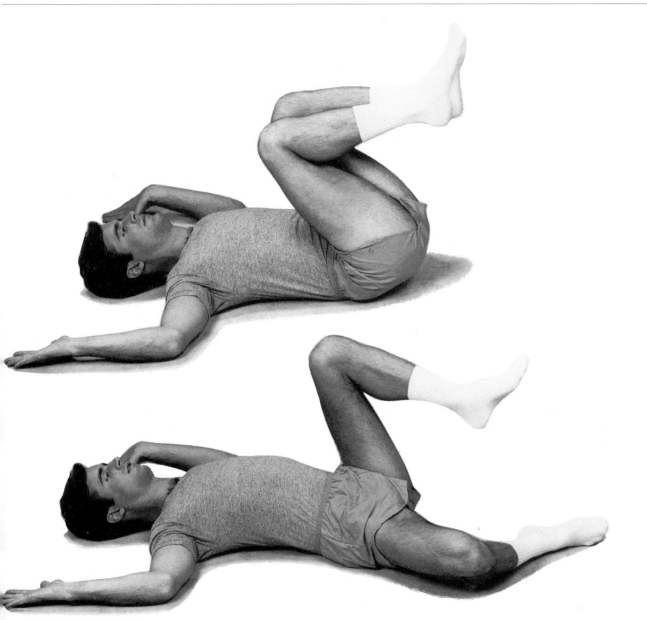

❏ Repeat as in Phase I.

NOTE: Every time you do this stretch, your body will be even more relaxed. Take advantage of this time to clear your mind and think beautiful, positive, wonderful thoughts. Transport yourself through your imagination to the place you'd like to go most . . . a desert island, an exhilarating mountaintop . . . you decide. Relax and enjoy it!

DON'TS

❏ **Do not tense or jerk your body.**

❏ **Do not rush through this stretch.**

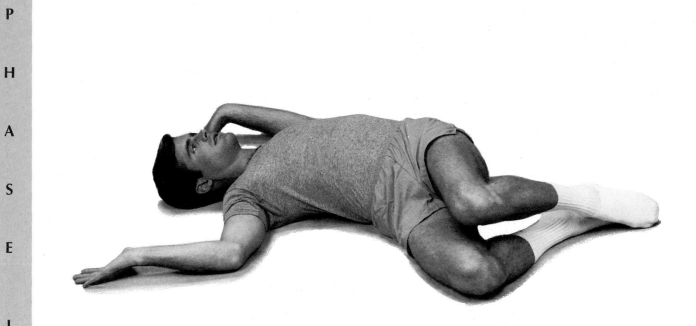

Hold for a count of . . .						
TO EACH SIDE						
1	2	3	4	DAY 5 60	DAY 6 60	DAY 7 60
DAY 8 60	DAY 9 60	10	11	12	13	14
15	16	17	18	19	20	21
22	23	24	25	26	27	28
29	30					

Neck to the Side

TECHNIQUE

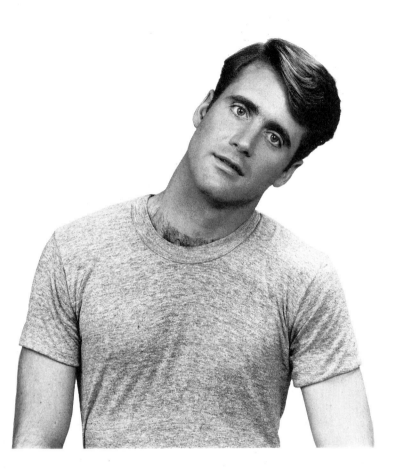

DON'TS

❏ Do not hunch or tense your shoulders.

❏ Do not make any jerky movements.

❏ Repeat as in Phase I.

Repetitions
TO EACH SIDE

1	2	3	4	DAY 5 1	DAY 6 1	DAY 7 1
DAY 8 1	DAY 9 1	10	11	12	13	14
15	16	17	18	19	20	21
22	23	24	25	26	27	28
29	30					

The Three-Quarter Neck Relaxer

TECHNIQUE

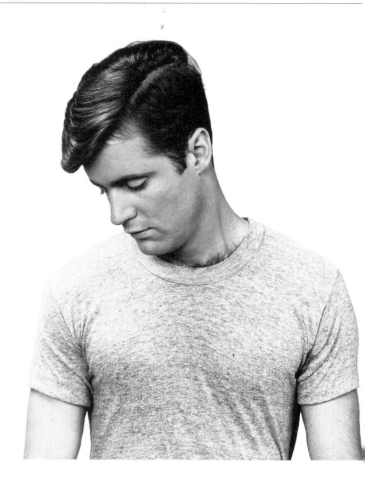

DON'TS

❏ **Do not force your head down.**

❏ **Do not tense your shoulders.**

Repeat as in Phase I.

NOTE: The more relaxed your shoulders are, the more of a stretch you will get. As you continue to stretch these muscles, tightness and tension will be released, giving you greater mobility.

Repetitions
TO EACH SIDE

1	2	3	4	DAY 5 1	DAY 6 1	DAY 7 1
DAY 8 1	DAY 9 1	10	11	12	13	14
15	16	17	18	19	20	21
22	23	24	25	26	27	28
29	30					

LEGS AND INNER THIGHS

Bend and Curl

TECHNIQUE

❑ Repeat as in Phase I, but this time raise your heels off the floor about one to two inches, keeping your legs apart, feet turned out slightly for balance. In addition, instead of lowering your body and curling up your pelvis just two times, now go down three times and back up three times. This again is one repetition.

NOTE: By now, you should be able to curl up your pelvis further. With even a sixteenth of an inch more, you'll feel an incredible difference. When lowering your body, you should try to keep your torso erect. However, when you start to curl up your pelvis, aiming your pubic bone more into the navel, your upper back will automatically start to round. Allow this to happen—it's a thrilling development—for now you are not only tightening your legs and inner thighs, but you're also getting a wonderful, tension-releasing stretch in your spine.

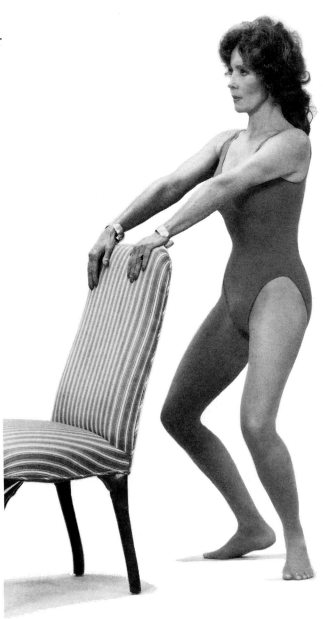

Don'ts

❏ **Do not stick out your buttocks or stomach.**

❏ **Do not allow your buttocks to drop lower than your knees.**

❏ **Do not let your heels drop to the floor.**

❏ **Do not tense your shoulders.**

Repetitions

1	2	3	4	DAY 5	DAY 6	DAY 7
				3	4	4
DAY 8	DAY 9	10	11	12	13	14
5	5					
15	16	17	18	19	20	21
22	23	24	25	26	27	28
29	30					

Plié and Balance

TECHNIQUE

❑ Repeat as in Phase I, but this time raise your heels two inches off the floor, keeping your legs apart, feet turned out slightly for balance. In *triple slow motion*, lower your body two inches and return to the starting position, with your knees bent, your heels off the floor.

Those of you with ballet training may recognize this movement. It is, indeed, a standard ballet plié that I have modified slightly. However, even if you have had ballet, you may find it difficult to do at first.

DON'TS

❏ **Do not stick out your buttocks or your stomach.**

❏ **Do not drop your heels, going down or coming back up.**

❏ **Do not tense your shoulders.**

Repetitions

1	2	3	4	DAY 5 5	DAY 6 7	DAY 7 9
DAY 8 10	DAY 9 10	10	11	12	13	14
15	16	17	18	19	20	21
22	23	24	25	26	27	28
29	30					

Up and Over

❑ Repeat as in Phase I, but this time try to straighten the knee of the raised leg. If you are able, try lifting your leg onto a higher "barre." (If you can't find a suitable higher surface, simply scoot the standing leg back further.) Remember to hold your elbows out to the sides to stretch between your shoulder blades. To come out of this position, bend the raised leg and gently take it down. Work both sides.

NOTE: If you are one of those people who has puffiness on the inside of the knees, simply rotating the raised leg when doing this exercise can help tighten it. For example, if your right leg is extended on your "barre," turn it to the right and this will extend the stretch to include the inside of the knee.

DON'TS

❏ **Do not lock either of your knees.**

❏ **Do not rest your hands on your knee.**

❏ **Do not make jerking movements with your neck or torso.**

❏ **Do not force the raised leg straight by pushing your leg or knee down with your hands.**

❏ **Do not tense your neck or shoulders.**

Repetitions
TO EACH SIDE

1	2	3	4	DAY 5 **25**	DAY 6 **30**	DAY 7 **35**
DAY 8 **40**	DAY 9 **40**	10	11	12	13	14
15	16	17	18	19	20	21
22	23	24	25	26	27	28
29	30					

Hamstring Stretch

TECHNIQUE

❏ Repeat as in Phase I, but this time hold on to your calf instead of your thigh, and extend your elbows even further out to the side to stretch between your shoulder blades. Try to straighten your leg if you can. Hold for a count of thirty before you begin your repetitions. Work both sides.

NOTE: As you become more proficient, you will be able to extend your elbows further and further out to the side. You will also be able to bring your legs closer and closer to your chin, but be patient—don't force it.

Don'ts

❏ Do not bounce.

❏ Do not force the raised leg forward by pulling it.

❏ Do not force the raised leg to straighten.

❏ Do not tense your neck.

Repetitions
TO EACH SIDE

1	2	3	4	DAY 5 30	DAY 6 35	DAY 7 40
DAY 8 45	DAY 9 50	10	11	12	13	14
15	16	17	18	19	20	21
22	23	24	25	26	27	28
29	30					

The Standing Stretch

TECHNIQUE

❏ Repeat as in Phase I, but this time, very gently, still resting your foot in your hand, curl up your pelvis. You will feel this stretch in the front-thigh muscle called the quadriceps. Work both sides.

NOTE: When you begin this exercise, you may find that, as you curl up your pelvis, the raised knee will move forward with the pelvis. Allow this to happen. Your muscles will stretch gradually and you will be able to lead your knee further to the back.

DON'Ts

❏ Do not let the foot of the bent leg touch your buttocks.

❏ Do not arch your back or stick out your stomach.

❏ Do not lock your elbows or the knee of the standing leg.

Hold for a count of . . .

TO EACH SIDE

1	2	3	4	DAY 5 30	DAY 6 30	DAY 7 35
DAY 8 40	DAY 9 40	10	11	12	13	14
15	16	17	18	19	20	21
22	23	24	25	26	27	28
29	30					

The Inner-Thigh Tightener

TECHNIQUE

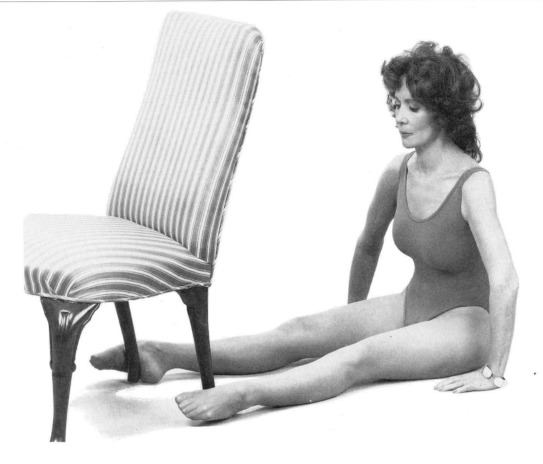

❑ Repeat as in Phase I, but this time try to straighten your legs.

NOTE: As your muscles gain strength, you will find that you can do this exercise sitting more erect, but it's very important to stay relaxed.

DON'TS

❑ Do not squeeze and release; hold steadily for the count.

❑ Do not tense your shoulders.

❑ Do not lock your knees.

Hold for a count of . . .

1	2	3	4	DAY 5 50	DAY 6 50	DAY 7 50
DAY 8 50	DAY 9 50	10	11	12	13	14
15	16	17	18	19	20	21
22	23	24	25	26	27	28
29	30					

BUTTOCKS, HIPS, AND OUTER THIGHS

Bringing Up the Rear

TECHNIQUE

❏ In front of a sofa or chair, sit on your left buttock with your left knee bent and resting comfortably on the floor in front of you, your heel several inches away from your body. Your right leg is out to the side, knee bent and even with your right hip, if possible. Your toes should be relaxed and pointing to the back. Rest your elbows and forearms on the seat of the chair or sofa and lean your torso over to the left. Lift your right leg so that your knee is a few inches off the floor, still trying to keep it even with your right hip. Gently, in *triple slow motion*, move your right knee one-sixteenth to one-quarter inch to the back, then return it even with the hip. After you have completed your repetitions, slowly lower it to the floor. If you find that your muscles are not strong enough to support this motion, or you cannot do it without leaning your torso forward or arching your lower back, then lean your torso even further to the left—as far as you need to. Once the buttock muscles are strong enough, you will be able to straighten up your torso gradually. Reverse and repeat the exercise to the other side.

NOTE: If you are raising your leg too high and aiming your knee upward, you will be working the front-thigh muscles more than your buttocks. Instead of compensating in this way, lean your torso further to the side or take a breather. This is a sign that the buttock muscles may be weak.

DON'TS

❑ **Do not stick out your buttocks.**

❑ **Do not tense any part of your body, especially your shoulders.**

❑ **Do not push out your stomach.**

❑ **Do not arch your back.**

Repetitions
TO EACH SIDE

1	2	3	4	DAY 5 30	DAY 6 35	DAY 7 40
DAY 8 45	DAY 9 50	10	11	12	13	14
15	16	17	18	19	20	21
22	23	24	25	26	27	28
29	30					

Out to the Side

TECHNIQUE

❑ Repeat as in Phase I, but this time take the extended leg directly out to the side, so that it is as even with your hip as possible. Try to straighten the extended leg so that your foot, knee, and hip are even, but do not force it. Lift your leg no more than six to eight inches off the floor. Work both sides.

NOTE: If your buttock muscles are not strong enough to support this motion, or you cannot do it without arching your back, lean as far over to the side opposite the extended leg as you need to, making sure that the lower back is stretched so that you don't put any pressure on it. Once your muscles are strong enough, you will be able to straighten your torso gradually and lift your leg with ease.

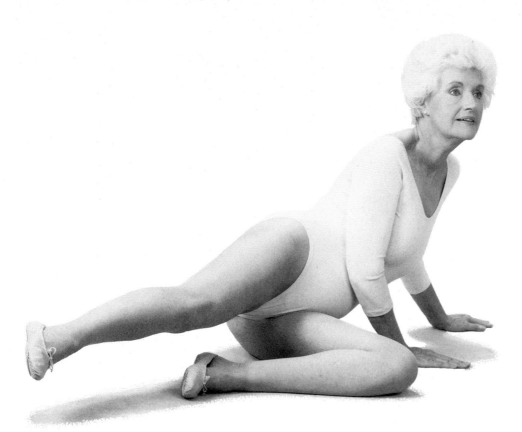

DON'TS

❏ Do not stick out your stomach.

❏ Do not arch your back.

❏ Do not tense your neck or shoulders

❏ Do not lock your knee.

Repetitions
TO EACH SIDE

1	2	3	4	DAY 5 30	DAY 6 35	DAY 7 40
DAY 8 45	DAY 9 50	10	11	12	13	14
15	16	17	18	19	20	21
22	23	24	25	26	27	28
29	30					

Pelvic Circles

TECHNIQUE

❏ Repeat as in Phase I, but this time bring your arms straight up over your head, clasp your hands and try to stretch your whole upper torso to the point where you can feel the stretch in your lower back. Then lower your body six inches, and continue as in Phase I.

NOTE: When you begin, do these motions in triple slow motion. As you become more adept, you can gradually increase your pace.

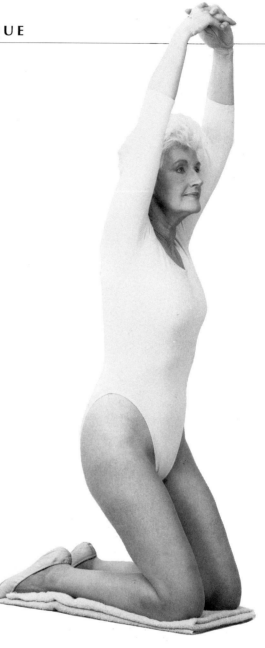

Repetitions
IN EACH DIRECTION

1	2	3	4	DAY 5	DAY 6	DAY 7
				3	3	3
DAY 8	DAY 9	10	11	12	13	14
3	3					
15	16	17	18	19	20	21
22	23	24	25	26	27	28
29	30					

DON'TS

❏ Do not arch your back.

❏ Do not stick out your stomach.

❏ Do not try to do too much too fast.

The Pelvic Dip

TECHNIQUE

DON'TS

❏ **Do not arch your back.**

❏ **Do not jerk up your pelvis.**

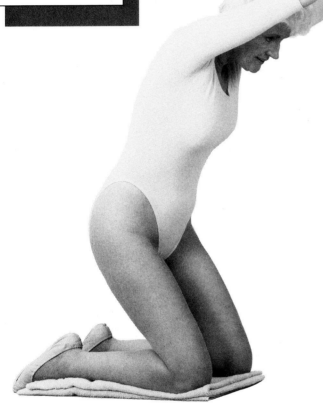

❏ From the starting position, stretch your arms and torso as in Phase I. Continue to stretch as you aim your buttocks toward your heels. Round and lean your torso forward while slowly lowering your buttocks, as if you were going to sit down. Aim toward your heels and make sure you do not arch your back. Lower yourself about six to eight inches, then tighten your buttock muscles and slowly curl up your pelvis. Return to the starting position using the strength of your thighs as in Phase I.

NOTE: As you become more adept at this exercise, you won't have to lean forward and will be able to keep your shoulders back even more as you come up.

Repetitions

1	2	3	4	DAY 5 3	DAY 6 3	DAY 7 3
DAY 8 3	DAY 9 3	10	11	12	13	14
15	16	17	18	19	20	21
22	23	24	25	26	27	28
29	30					

The Front-Thigh Stretch

TECHNIQUE

❏ Repeat as in Phase I, but this time, instead of making fists with your hands, try to place your palms on the floor in back of you.

NOTE: *This movement will seem easier if you try to stay conscious of relaxing your entire body as you do it.*

DON'TS

❏ Do not arch your back or stick out your stomach.

❏ Do not tense your body.

❏ Do not hunch your shoulders.

Hold for a count of . . .

1	2	3	4	DAY 5 20	DAY 6 20	DAY 7 20
DAY 8 20	DAY 9 20	10	11	12	13	14
15	16	17	18	19	20	21
22	23	24	25	26	27	28
29	30					

The Crossover

TECHNIQUE

❏ Repeat as in Phase I, but as you take your knee over, bring your foot with it, in front of your extended leg. Let your leg dangle, as close to the floor as gravity pulls it. Then, in *triple slow motion*, move your right knee no more than one sixteenth of an inch toward the floor and back. Work both sides.

NOTE: Be sure that your shoulders and elbows do not come off the floor. You will get the greatest benefit from this stretch, especially in the area of the lower back, if you concentrate on keeping your shoulders and elbows down, rather than bringing your knee down.

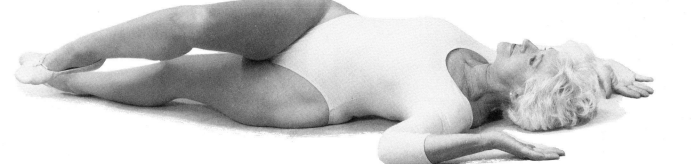

DON'TS

❏ Do not lift your shoulders off the floor.

❏ Do not bring your elbows off the floor.

❏ Do not turn your head to either side.

❏ Do not jerk the bent knee.

❏ Do not force the stretch.

Repetitions
TO EACH SIDE

1	2	3	4	DAY 5 15	DAY 6 20	DAY 7 25
DAY 8 30	DAY 9 30	10	11	12	13	14
15	16	17	18	19	20	21
22	23	24	25	26	27	28
29	30					

PHASE III

This is a thrilling time. You've learned to appreciate what an impact those tiny one-sixteenth-of-an-inch motions can have on your stomach, legs, hips, and buttocks. With all this progress, it's important to stay alert to the signals your body sends you. Is it telling you to slow down? Is it telling you it's capable of more and ready to move on? Remember to take the time to appreciate the magnificent way you are put together. This is the time students start to get excited about their bodies and want to show them off! Even if you don't think you see dramatic changes yet, friends may comment that you look "different"—*good* different.

WARM-UPS

The Underarm Tightener

TECHNIQUE

❏ Repeat as in Phase I, but this time try the exercise standing erect, your feet a hip-width apart, your knees bent. Each day you do this exercise, try to keep your arms as high as possible, in back of you, with your shoulders and head held back.

NOTE: When you first attempt this exercise, you may find that your head and shoulders round forward and that it is difficult to keep your buttocks from sticking out. As you become stronger, you will be able to stand more and more erect.

DON'TS

❏ Do not jerk your arms back and forth.

❏ Do not arch your back or stick out your stomach.

❏ Do not lock your elbows.

❏ Do not tense your shoulders.

❏ Do not lock your knees.

Repetitions

1	2	3	4	5	6	7
8	9	DAY 10 **50**	DAY 11 **60**	DAY 12 **70**	DAY 13 **80**	DAY 14 **90**
DAY 15 **100**	DAY 16 **100**	17	18	19	20	21
22	23	24	25	26	27	28
29	30					

The Waist Away

TECHNIQUE

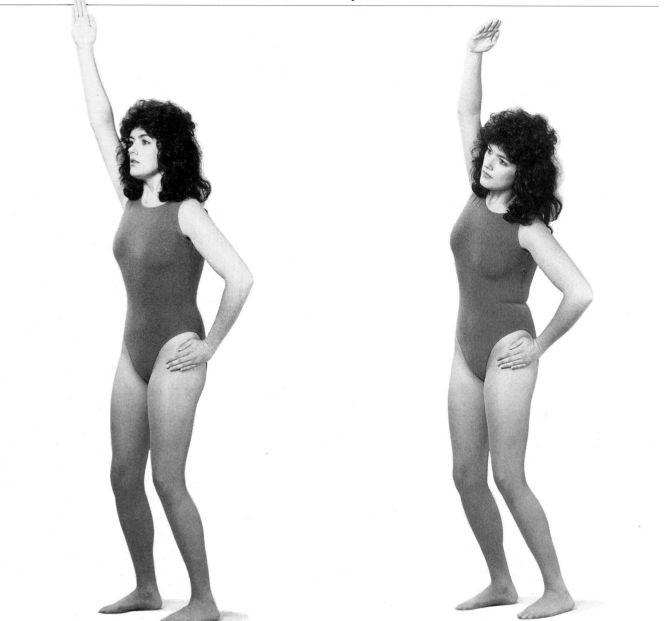

❑ Repeat as in Phase II, but this time, instead of resting your arm on a "barre," support yourself by placing your hand just below your hip, your elbow pointing straight out to the side, if possible, and straighten your knees a bit. Slowly stretch your other arm upward, palm facing inward. Stretch up and over to the side, trying to move your upper body and arm together. You may bend slightly forward if necessary. Continue as in Phase II.

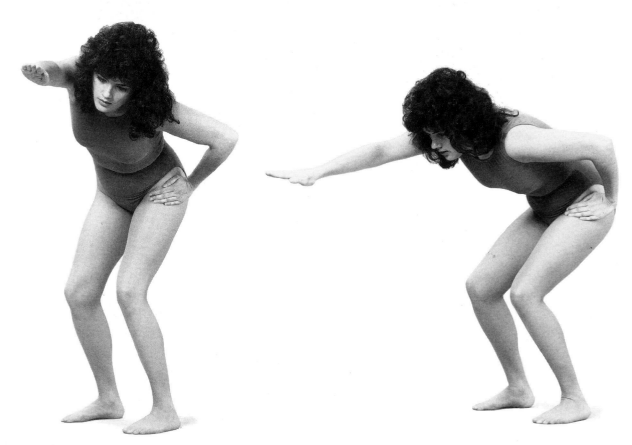

❏ To reverse sides, keep your hand on your hip and bend your knees even more. Continue to stretch the right arm over, and continue around to the front, slowly extending your arm down and then over to the right side in a slow sweeping movement. Tighten your buttocks, curl up your pelvis, and slowly straighten your spine, vertebra by vertebra, as you lower the arm. Repeat the exercise on the left side. When you have completed the left side, come out of the exercise as above.

NOTE: *At first you may have trouble keeping your arm fully extended and curling your pelvis up.*

DON'TS

❏ **Do not bounce.**

❏ **Do not tense your shoulders or neck.**

❏ **Do not arch your lower back or stick out your stomach.**

❏ **Do not let your resting elbow point forward or backward.**

❏ **Do not lock your knees.**

Repetitions
TO EACH SIDE

1	2	3	4	5	6	7
8	9	**DAY 10** 50	**DAY 11** 60	**DAY 12** 70	**DAY 13** 80	**DAY 14** 90
DAY 15 100	**DAY 16** 100	17	18	19	20	21
22	23	24	25	26	27	28
29	30					

The Neck Stretch

TECHNIQUE

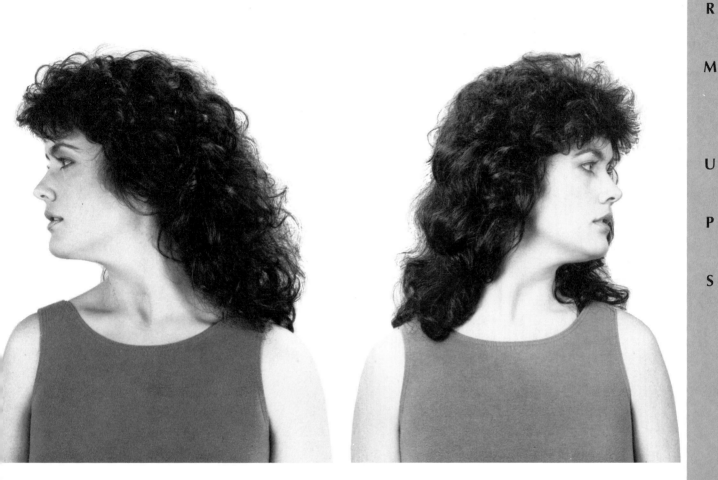

❏ Repeat as in Phase II, but this time curl up your pelvis at the same time as far as you can, to stretch your spine.

Repetitions
TO EACH SIDE

1	2	3	4	5	6	7
8	9	DAY 10 5	DAY 11 5	DAY 12 5	DAY 13 5	DAY 14 5
DAY 15 5	DAY 16 5	17	18	19	20	21
22	23	24	25	26	27	28
29	30					

DON'TS

❏ Do not turn your body or rotate your shoulders.

❏ Do not lock your knees.

❏ Do not tense your shoulders.

❏ Do not stick out your buttocks or stomach.

The Neck Roll

TECHNIQUE

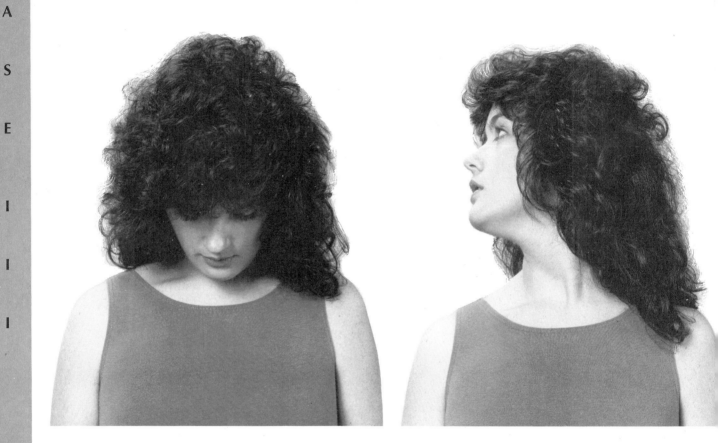

❏ Repeat as in Phase II, but this time curl up your pelvis at the same time, as far as you can, to stretch your spine.

Repetitions
TO EACH SIDE

1	2	3	4	5	6	7
8	9	DAY 10 5	DAY 11 5	DAY 12 5	DAY 13 5	DAY 14 5
DAY 15 5	DAY 16 5	17	18	19	20	21
22	23	24	25	26	27	28
29	30					

DON'TS

❏ Do not make any sharp or sudden movements.

❏ Do not hunch or tense your shoulders.

❏ Do not tense your jaw.

❏ Do not lock your knees.

❏ Do not stick out your buttocks or stomach.

THE STOMACH

The Bent-Knee Reach

TECHNIQUE

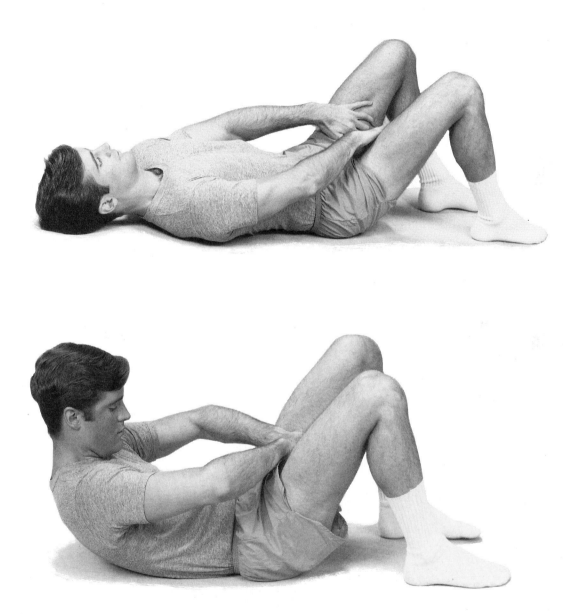

❏ Repeat as in Phase II, but this time keep your feet flat on the floor and hold on to your *inner* thighs with all your might. Still holding on, take your elbows out to the sides of your body as far as possible, then point them upward as far as possible before you gently round your head and shoulders off the floor, aiming your nose into your chest. Complete as in Phase II.

NOTE: Pay particular attention to your starting position. Done correctly, this exercise builds muscle strength very quickly, and this will enable you to take your elbows out more and up higher, which in turn lets you round more and strengthen faster.

DON'TS

❑ **Do not rock your entire body back and forth.**

❑ **Do not tighten your buttocks.**

❑ **Do not bounce your head or aim it up toward the ceiling.**

❑ **Do not hold in your stomach muscles.**

❑ **Do not hold your breath.**

❑ **Do not lift your head first.**

Repetitions

1	2	3	4	5	6	7
8	9	DAY 10 **50**	DAY 11 **60**	DAY 12 **70**	DAY 13 **80**	DAY 14 **90**
DAY 15 **100**	DAY 16 **100**	17	18	19	20	21
22	23	24	25	26	27	28
29	30					

Single-Leg Raises

TECHNIQUE

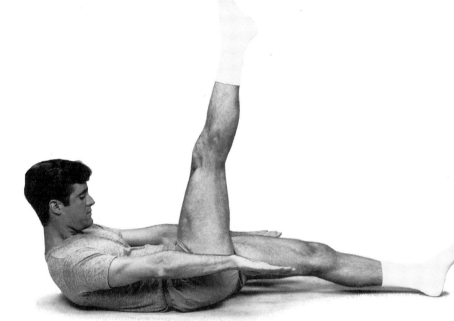

❏ Repeat as in Phase II, but this time try to straighten the raised leg as much as possible and try to straighten the other leg along the floor in front of you. Relax your legs and toes. When you release your arms to your sides, your shoulders may drop toward the floor a little. If you find this too difficult at first, keep holding on to your leg until you build up enough strength. Work both sides.

NOTE: Try to keep the raised leg as perpendicular to the floor as possible. If your stomach muscles aren't strong enough and you start to lower it toward the floor, the weight of your leg will activate your hip flexors, putting pressure on your lower back.

Repetitions
TO EACH SIDE

1	2	3	4	5	6	7
8	9	DAY 10 **50**	DAY 11 **60**	DAY 12 **70**	DAY 13 **80**	DAY 14 **90**
DAY 15 **100**	DAY 16 **100**	17	18	19	20	21
22	23	24	25	26	27	28
29	30					

Double-Leg Raises

TECHNIQUE

❏ Repeat as in Phase II, trying to straighten your legs even more.

NOTE: Learn to completely relax your legs. You do not have to tense them to hold them up.

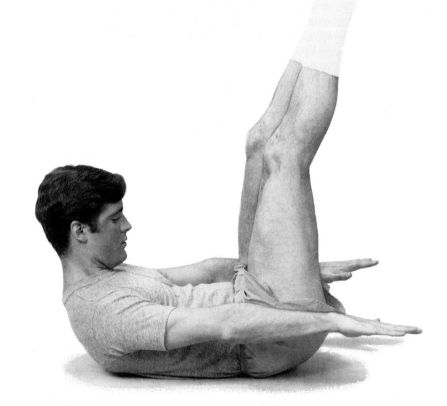

DON'TS

❏ Do not lift up your legs without bending your knees first.

❏ Do not tense your legs, knees, or toes.

❏ Do not jerk your neck.

❏ Do not tense your neck or shoulders.

❏ Do not rock your body back and forth.

Repetitions

1	2	3	4	5	6	7
8	9	DAY 10 **50**	DAY 11 **60**	DAY 12 **70**	DAY 13 **80**	DAY 14 **90**
DAY 15 **100**	DAY 16 **100**	17	18	19	20	21
22	23	24	25	26	27	28
29	30					

Both Legs Over

TECHNIQUE

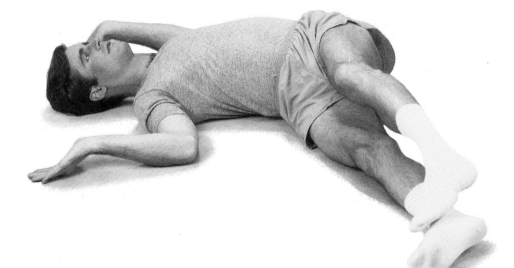

❏ Repeat as in Phase II, but this time, after you take your knees over to the side, try to straighten your legs—only as far as you comfortably can—before you hold for the count.

NOTE: Remember to keep both shoulders on the floor, and try to relax your entire body.

DON'TS

❏ Do not tense or jerk your body.

❏ Do not rush through this stretch.

❏ Do not force the stretch.

Hold for a count of . . .
TO EACH SIDE

1	2	3	4	5	6	7
8	9	DAY 10 **50**	DAY 11 **50**	DAY 12 **50**	DAY 13 **50**	DAY 14 **50**
DAY 15 **50**	DAY 16 **50**	17	18	19	20	21
22	23	24	25	26	27	28
29	30					

Neck to the Side

TECHNIQUE

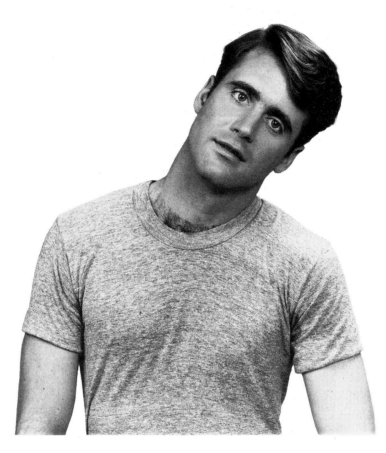

❑ Repeat as in Phase I.

NOTE: As your muscles continue to stretch, you will be able to lower your head even closer to your shoulders.

DON'TS

❑ Do not hunch or tense your shoulders.

❑ Do not make any jerky movements.

Repetitions
TO EACH SIDE

1	2	3	4	5	6	7
8	9	DAY 10 1	DAY 11 1	DAY 12 1	DAY 13 1	DAY 14 1
DAY 15 1	DAY 16 1	17	18	19	20	21
22	23	24	25	26	27	28
29	30					

Three-Quarter Neck Relaxer

TECHNIQUE

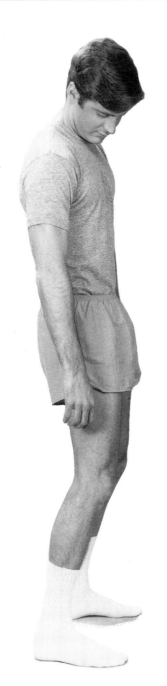

❏ Repeat as in Phase I, standing. Before beginning the neck movements, bend your knees, tighten your buttocks and curl up your pelvis to stretch your spine.

DON'TS

❏ **Do not force your head down.**

❏ **Do not tense your shoulders.**

❏ **Do not lock your knees.**

Repetitions
TO EACH SIDE

1	2	3	4	5	6	7
8	9	DAY 10 **1**	DAY 11 **1**	DAY 12 **1**	DAY 13 **1**	DAY 14 **1**
DAY 15 **1**	DAY 16 **1**	17	18	19	20	21
22	23	24	25	26	27	28
29	30					

LEGS AND INNER THIGHS

Bend and Curl

TECHNIQUE

❏ Repeat as in Phase II, but raise your heels off the floor three to four inches and move your feet together so that your heels touch. Your feet will be slightly turned out.

NOTE: With your heels off the floor, at first you may find it difficult to curl up your pelvis. You will gradually get better at this movement, and this will start to stretch your spine and work your inner thighs more. Your balance will also improve, and you won't feel that you need to clutch the "barre" using every muscle in your body.

DON'TS

❏ Do not stick out your buttocks or stomach.

❏ Do not allow your buttocks to drop lower than your knees.

❏ Do not let your heels drop to the floor.

❏ Do not tense your shoulders.

Repetitions

1	2	3	4	5	6	7
8	9	DAY 10 5	DAY 11 5	DAY 12 6	DAY 13 6	DAY 14 7
DAY 15 7	DAY 16 7	17	18	19	20	21
22	23	24	25	26	27	28
29	30					

Plié and Balance

TECHNIQUE

❏ Repeat as in Phase II, but this time raise your heels two to three inches off the floor and then move your feet together so that your heels touch. Turn out your feet so that your knees are over your toes. This time, in *triple slow motion,* lower your body four inches.

NOTE: You will improve as you continue to do this exercise, and will soon be able to perform it keeping your shoulders relaxed and your spine straight.

DON'TS

❏ **Do not stick out your buttocks or your stomach.**

❏ **Do not drop your heels, going down or coming up.**

❏ **Do not tense your shoulders.**

Repetitions

1	2	3	4	5	6	7
8	9	**DAY 10** **10**	**DAY 11** **10**	**DAY 12** **11**	**DAY 13** **12**	**DAY 14** **13**
DAY 15 **14**	**DAY 16** **15**	17	18	19	20	21
22	23	24	25	26	27	28
29	30					

Up and Over

TECHNIQUE

❏ Repeat as in Phase II, using a higher "barre" (but only as high as comfortable) and continuing to try to straighten your raised leg. Concentrate on letting your entire body melt. Work both sides.

NOTE: To make your "barre" higher, all you have to do is put a thick book (like a dictionary) or a firm throw pillow on top of what you were using. Just be sure it won't slip. You may also simply choose another piece of furniture to use.

At first it may be difficult to keep your standing foot facing front. In order to maintain your balance, you may have to turn the foot a little to the side. As you get better at this stretch, you will be able to keep it facing forward, rather than turned out.

Don'ts

❑ Do not lock either of your knees.

❑ Do not rest your hands on your knees.

❑ Do not make jerking movements with your neck or torso.

❑ Do not force the raised leg straight by pushing your leg or knee down with your hands.

❑ Do not tense your neck or shoulders.

❑ Do not attempt a greater height than is comfortable.

Repetitions
TO EACH SIDE

1	2	3	4	5	6	7
8	9	**DAY 10** 40	**DAY 11** 45	**DAY 12** 45	**DAY 13** 50	**DAY 14** 50
DAY 15 50	**DAY 16** 50	17	18	19	20	21
22	23	24	25	26	27	28
29	30					

Hamstring Stretch

TECHNIQUE

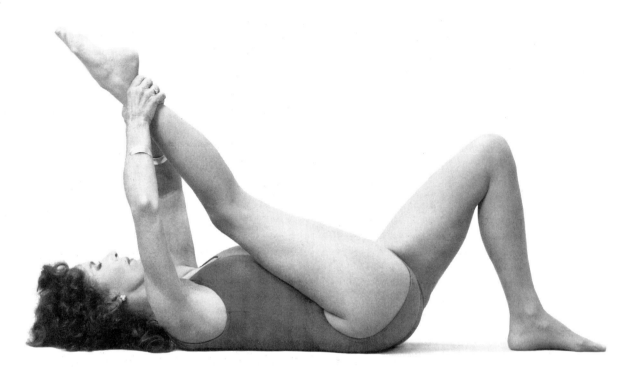

❏ Repeat as in Phase II, but this time, if you can straighten your leg, hold on to your ankle for more of a stretch. If you are not stretched enough for this, continue to hold on to your calf. Try to straighten your raised leg even more toward your chest. Work both sides.

NOTE: If your muscles are stretched enough, you can try to flex the toes on your raised foot. This will stretch your calf muscle as well.

DON'TS

❏ Do not bounce.

❏ Do not force the raised leg forward by pulling it.

❏ Do not force the raised leg to straighten.

❏ Do not tense your neck.

Repetitions
TO EACH SIDE

1	2	3	4	5	6	7
8	9	**DAY 10** 50	**DAY 11** 55	**DAY 12** 60	**DAY 13** 65	**DAY 14** 70
DAY 15 75	**DAY 16** 75	17	18	19	20	21
22	23	24	25	26	27	28
29	30					

The Standing Stretch

TECHNIQUE

❑ Repeat as in Phase II. Curl up your pelvis and very gently try to take the knee back so that both knees are more or less even. Work both sides.

NOTE: The more stretched the thigh becomes, the more you will be able to curl up the pelvis while keeping the knee aimed into the floor. This stretches these muscles even more!

DON'TS

❑ **Do not let the foot of the bent leg touch your buttocks.**

❑ **Do not arch your back or stick out your stomach.**

❑ **Do not lock your elbows or the knee of the standing leg.**

Hold for a count of . . .
TO EACH SIDE

1	2	3	4	5	6	7
8	9	**DAY 10** **40**	**DAY 11** **45**	**DAY 12** **45**	**DAY 13** **50**	**DAY 14** **50**
DAY 15 **50**	**DAY 16** **50**	17	18	19	20	21
22	23	24	25	26	27	28
29	30					

The Inner-Thigh Tightener

TECHNIQUE

❏ Repeat as in Phase II, lifting your feet one to four inches off the floor, as is comfortable, and continuing to try to keep your legs straight.

NOTE: *When doing this exercise, if your feet keep slipping, try removing your socks. Bare feet won't slide as much.*

DON'TS

❏ Do not squeeze and release; hold steadily for the count.

❏ Do not tense your shoulders.

❏ Do not lock your knees.

Hold for a count of . . .

1	2	3	4	5	6	7
8	9	DAY 10 **75**	DAY 11 **75**	DAY 12 **75**	DAY 13 **75**	DAY 14 **75**
DAY 15 **75**	DAY 16 **75**	17	18	19	20	21
22	23	24	25	26	27	28
29	30					

BUTTOCKS, HIPS, AND OUTER THIGHS

Bringing Up the Rear

TECHNIQUE

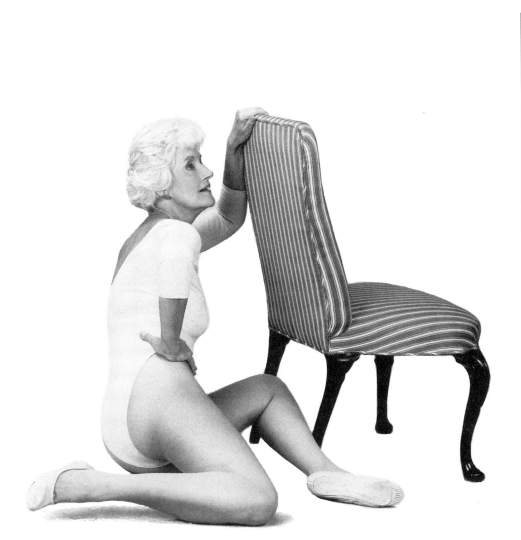

> **DON'TS**
>
> ❏ **Do not stick out your buttocks.**
>
> ❏ **Do not tense any part of your body, especially your shoulders.**
>
> ❏ **Do not push out your stomach.**
>
> ❏ **Do not arch your back.**

❏ Position yourself as in Phase II, this time holding on to a "barre" (a sofa or chair, a table, or anything else strong enough to support you) with your left hand. Place your right hand on your right hip.

❏ Rotate the right hip forward, rolling it over as far as it will go with your right hand, so that both hips are even with each other and facing forward. Your right foot *should* come off the floor, higher than the knee. If it doesn't, lift it up with your right hand.

❏ Trying not to let your hip roll back, put your right hand on the "barre." Leaning over to the opposite side as far as you need to, lift your right knee no more than four inches off the floor, keeping the knee even with your right hip. Keeping your foot higher than your knee, gently move your knee one-sixteenth to one-quarter inch back, then return. Do not let your knee come forward more than it did in the starting position. After you have completed your repetitions, slowly lower your leg to the floor. Reverse and repeat to the other side.

NOTE: Work up to the required number of repetitions by breaking it up into sets and switching from side to side, or taking breathers, if you have to.

Repetitions
TO EACH SIDE

1	2	3	4	5	6	7
8	9	DAY 10 50	DAY 11 55	DAY 12 60	DAY 13 65	DAY 14 70
DAY 15 75	DAY 16 75	17	18	19	20	21
22	23	24	25	26	27	28
29	30					

Out to the Side

TECHNIQUE

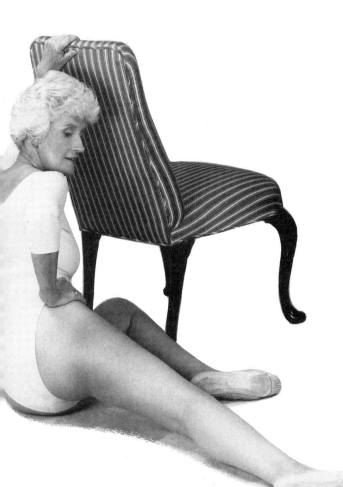

❏ Position yourself as in Phase II, but this time sit in front of and hold on to your "barre" with your left hand, and place your foot farther from your body. Using your right hand, gently rotate your right hip forward. Then grasp the "barre" with both hands, lean over to the side if you have to in order to lift your leg from one to three inches, and continue as in Phase II, straightening your working leg as far as you can. Work both sides.

DON'TS

❏ Do not stick out your stomach.

❏ Do not arch your back.

❏ Do not tense your neck or shoulders.

❏ Do not lock your knees.

NOTE: *Remember to take your leg directly out to the side, in line with your hip. It is common tendency to want to take the leg forward, but this will not get the results you want.*

Repetitions
TO EACH SIDE

1	2	3	4	5	6	7
8	9	DAY 10 **50**	DAY 11 **55**	DAY 12 **60**	DAY 13 **65**	DAY 14 **70**
DAY 15 **75**	DAY 16 **75**	17	18	19	20	21
22	23	24	25	26	27	28
29	30					

Pelvic Circles

Technique

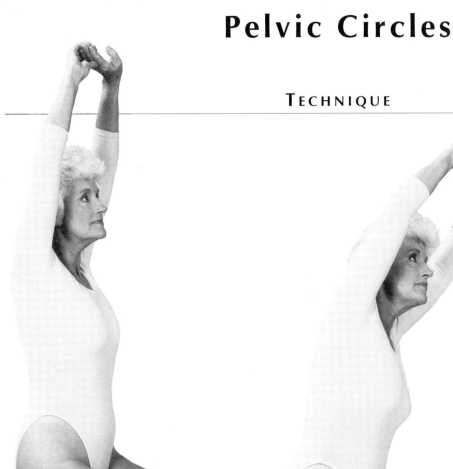

❏ Knees together, sit back on your heels, keeping your spine straight. Bring your arms over your head as in Phase II. Now, lift your body straight up about four inches off your heels, or higher if you have to. Continue to rotate your pelvis as in Phase I. Repeat in the opposite direction.

NOTE: It is important to remember to work at your own pace, taking breathers whenever you need them.

DON'TS

❏ Do not arch your back.

❏ Do not stick out your stomach.

❏ Do not try too much too fast.

Repetitions
IN EACH DIRECTION

1	2	3	4	5	6	7
8	9	DAY 10 **4**	DAY 11 **4**	DAY 12 **4**	DAY 13 **4**	DAY 14 **4**
DAY 15 **4**	DAY 16 **4**	17	18	19	20	21
22	23	24	25	26	27	28
29	30					

The Pelvic Dip

TECHNIQUE

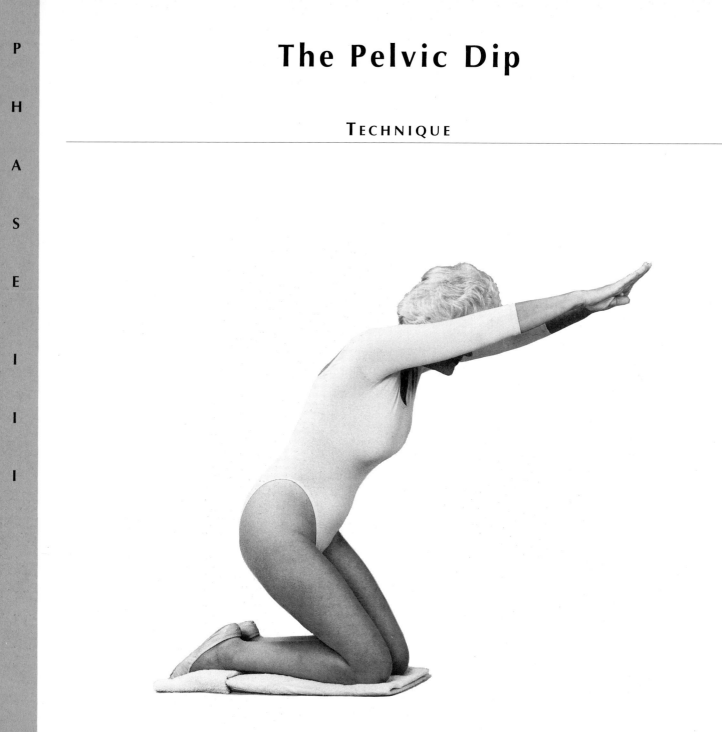

❏ Repeat as in Phase II, but with your knees together. Lower your body eight to ten inches.

NOTE: As you become more adept at this exercise, your movements will become more fluid. You will be able to keep your knees together easily and learn to relax your calf muscles.

DON'TS

❏ **Do not arch your back.**

❏ **Do not jerk up your pelvis.**

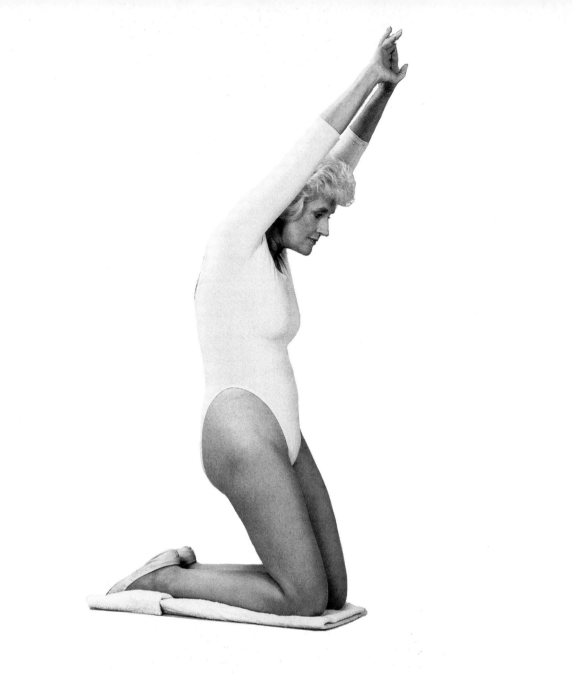

Repetitions

1	2	3	4	5	6	7
8	9	DAY 10 4	DAY 11 4	DAY 12 4	DAY 13 4	DAY 14 4
DAY 15 4	DAY 16 4	17	18	19	20	21
22	23	24	25	26	27	28
29	30					

The Front-Thigh Stretch

TECHNIQUE

❏ Repeat as in Phase II. When you have stretched enough to feel a slight pull in the front of your thighs, curl up your pelvis even more and lift your buttocks off your heels, no more than one inch at first. Hold this position for the count.

❏ Relax buttocks and gently return to the starting position, sitting on your heels. Relax your entire body.

DON'TS

❏ Do not arch your back or stick out your stomach.

❏ Do not allow your head to drop back.

❏ Do not tense your body.

❏ Do not hunch your shoulders or tense your neck.

Hold for a count of . . .

1	2	3	4	5	6	7
8	9	DAY 10 30	DAY 11 30	DAY 12 30	DAY 13 30	DAY 14 30
DAY 15 30	DAY 16 30	17	18	19	20	21
22	23	24	25	26	27	28
29	30					

The Crossover

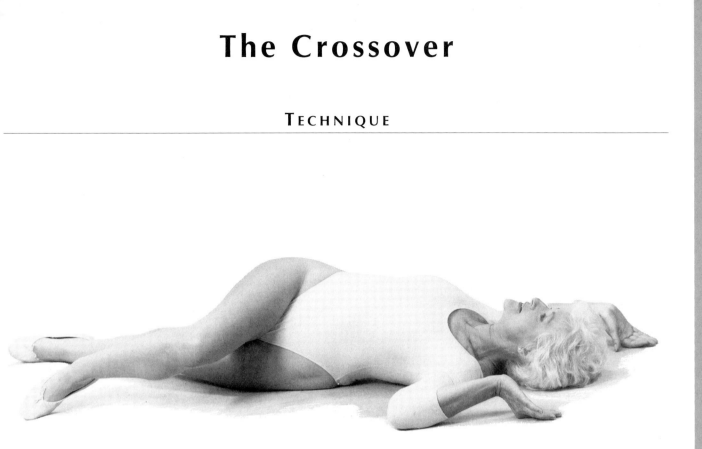

❑ Repeat as in Phase II, but try to touch your right toe to the floor. Continue as in Phase II, moving your right knee one sixteenth of an inch closer to the floor and back. Work both sides.

NOTE: As your muscles begin to stretch, you will enjoy doing this exercise more and more—I promise!

Repetitions
TO EACH SIDE

1	2	3	4	5	6	7
8	9	**DAY 10** 30	**DAY 11** 35	**DAY 12** 35	**DAY 13** 40	**DAY 14** 40
DAY 15 45	**DAY 16** 45	17	18	19	20	21
22	23	24	25	26	27	28
29	30					

DON'TS

❑ Do not lift your shoulders off the floor.

❑ Do not bring your elbows off the floor.

❑ Do not turn your head to either side.

❑ Do not jerk the bent knee.

❑ Do not force the stretch.

P H A S E
IV

You are now entering the final, most intense phase of the Callanetics Countdown. At last you're starting to work at peak capacity, and that's what brings about the most dramatic changes in your body. If you're going so strong that you begin to find these exercises too easy, even with the maximum number of repetitions, here are some modifications you can make.

Stomach: Round up even more.

Legs and inner thighs: Curl up more, increase the number of repetitions, and do the exercises at a slower pace.

Buttocks, hips, and outer thighs: Straighten your torso. Do more repetitions. Increase in increments of ten.

At the end of this book, you'll find some suggestions about how to keep Callanetics a regular part of your life, no matter how busy you get. In the meantime, enjoy the mental and physical strength you've gained, and the wonderful new way your body works. You've got it—now flaunt it.

WARM-UPS

The Underarm Tightener

TECHNIQUE

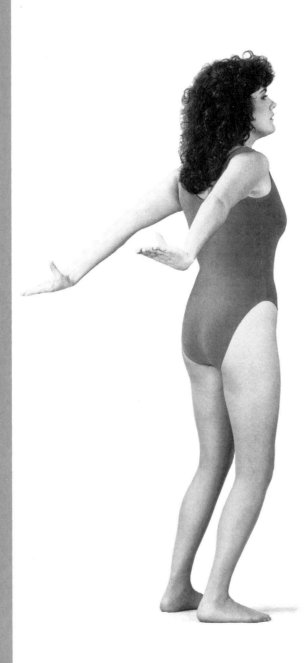

❏ Repeat as in Phase III, this time tightening your buttocks and curling up your pelvis, your knees only slightly bent. Try to hold your arms up even higher than before.

NOTE: The stronger your muscles get, the more you will be able to curl up your pelvis. You will also be able to hold your arms straighter, and your elbows won't bend. Because you will be able to rotate your arms and turn your wrists and hands further, you will be able to hold your arms higher while standing straight, and this will work your muscles even deeper and loosen the area between your shoulder blades even more.

Don'ts

❏ Do not jerk your arms back and forth.

❏ Do not arch your back or stick out your stomach.

❏ Do not lock your elbows.

❏ Do not tense your shoulders.

❏ Do not lock your knees.

Repetitions

1	2	3	4	5	6	7
8	9	10	11	12	13	14
15	16	DAY 17 75	DAY 18 85	DAY 19 100	DAY 20 100	DAY 21 100
DAY 22 100	DAY 23 100	DAY 24 100	DAY 25 100	DAY 26 100	DAY 27 100	DAY 28 100
DAY 29 100	DAY 30 100					

The Waist Away

TECHNIQUE

❏ Repeat as in Phase III, standing straight and tightening your buttocks and curling up the pelvis even more before you start reaching over to the side. Try to hold your extended arm by your ear. Work both sides.

NOTE: As your muscles get stronger, you will find that you can curl up your pelvis and bend over to the side even more. You will gradually be able to straighten your legs, still keeping them relaxed, and you will be able to keep your arm straight and by your ear. You will also become even more conscious of the wonderful stretch in your spine.

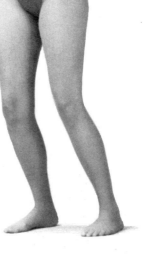

DON'TS

❏ Do not bounce.

❏ Do not tense your shoulders or neck.

❏ Do not arch your lower back or stick out your stomach.

❏ Do not let your resting elbow point forward or backward.

❏ Do not lock your knees.

Repetitions
TO EACH SIDE

1	2	3	4	5	6	7
8	9	10	11	12	13	14
15	16	DAY 17 75	DAY 18 85	DAY 19 100	DAY 20 100	DAY 21 100
DAY 22 100	DAY 23 100	DAY 24 100	DAY 25 100	DAY 26 100	DAY 27 100	DAY 28 100
DAY 29 100	DAY 30 100					

The Neck Stretch

TECHNIQUE

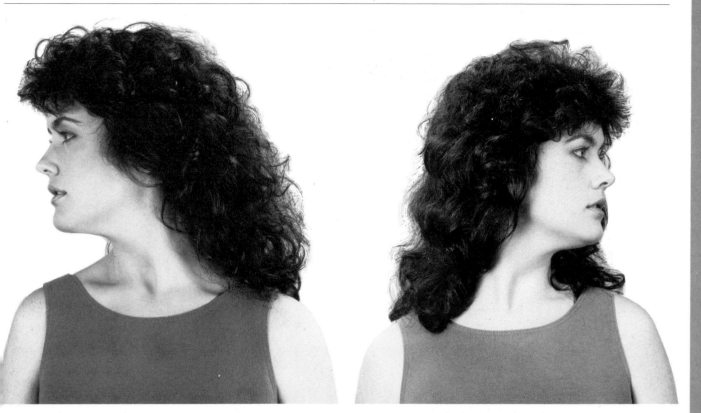

❑ Repeat as in Phase III.

NOTE: As your muscles relax even more, you will be able to curl up your pelvis more to stretch your spine and you won't have to bend your knees as much.

DON'TS

❑ **Do not turn your body or rotate your shoulders.**

❑ **Do not lock your knees.**

❑ **Do not tense your neck or shoulders.**

❑ **Do not stick out your buttocks or stomach.**

Repetitions
TO EACH SIDE

1	2	3	4	5	6	7
8	9	10	11	12	13	14
15	16	DAY 17 5	DAY 18 5	DAY 19 5	DAY 20 5	DAY 21 5
DAY 22 5	DAY 23 5	DAY 24 5	DAY 25 5	DAY 26 5	DAY 27 5	DAY 28 5
DAY 29 5	DAY 30 5					

The Neck Roll

TECHNIQUE

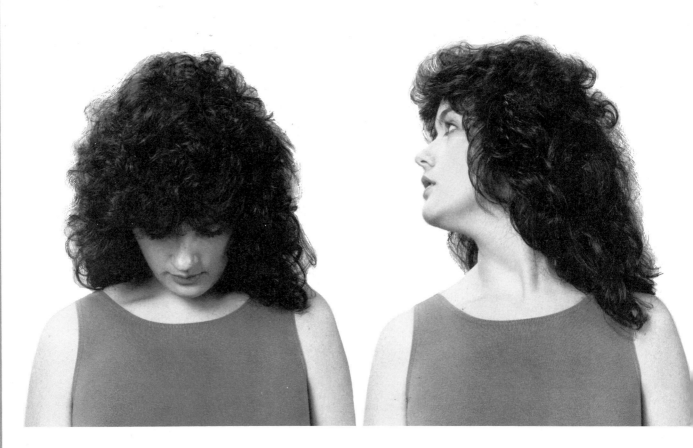

❏ Repeat as in Phase III, trying to curl up your pelvis even more, without bending your knees as much.

DON'TS

❏ Do not make any harsh or sudden movements.

❏ Do not hunch or tense your shoulders.

❏ Do not tense your jaw.

❏ Do not lock your knees.

❏ Do not stick out your stomach or arch your back.

Repetitions
TO EACH SIDE

1	2	3	4	5	6	7
8	9	10	11	12	13	14
15	16	DAY 17 5	DAY 18 5	DAY 19 5	DAY 20 5	DAY 21 5
DAY 22 5	DAY 23 5	DAY 24 5	DAY 25 5	DAY 26 5	DAY 27 5	DAY 28 5
DAY 29 5	DAY 30 5					

THE STOMACH

The Bent-Knee Reach

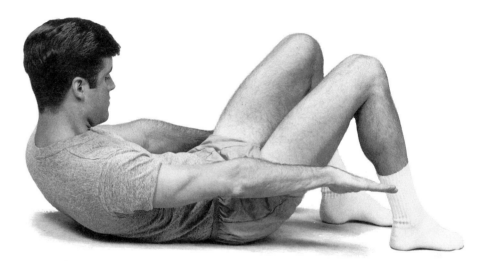

❏ Repeat as in Phase III, but when you can't round any more, release your hands and extend your arms straight out alongside your legs, so that they are parallel to the floor. Try to keep your legs loose and relaxed.

NOTE: As you learn to round up even more, this will gently stretch your neck and the area between your shoulder blades, releasing tension in the back and letting you focus on working the stomach muscles only. As you learn to relax, the rest of your body will feel like a rag doll. In addition, as your neck muscles stretch further, you may feel the muscles along the sides of your neck for a session or two. These are the muscles that make your neck look long and regal.

DON'TS

❏ **Do not rock your entire body back and forth.**

❏ **Do not tighten your buttocks.**

❏ **Do not bounce your head or aim it toward the ceiling.**

❏ **Do not hold in your stomach muscles.**

❏ **Do not hold your breath.**

❏ **Do not lift just your head first.**

❏ **Do not move just your arms.**

Repetitions

1	2	3	4	5	6	7
8	9	10	11	12	13	14
15	16	DAY 17 100	DAY 18 100	DAY 19 100	DAY 20 100	DAY 21 100
DAY 22 100	DAY 23 100	DAY 24 100	DAY 25 100	DAY 26 100	DAY 27 100	DAY 28 100
DAY 29 100	DAY 30 100					

Single-Leg Raises

TECHNIQUE

❏ Repeat as in Phase III, this time trying to round up even more and raising the extended leg several inches off the floor. Try to keep it perfectly straight and relaxed. Remember, move only one-sixteenth to one-quarter inch. Work both sides.

NOTE: As you continue to get stronger, you will be able to round your nose even more into your rib cage, and this will work your stomach muscles even more.

DON'TS

❏ Do not tense your toes, knees, or legs.

❏ Do not bring the raised leg toward your head, but, rather, round your body toward your leg.

❏ Do not rock your body back and forth.

❏ Do not jerk up your head.

❏ Do not aim your torso toward the ceiling.

❏ Do not tense your stomach.

❏ Do not forcibly tighten your buttocks.

❏ Do not move only your hands and arms.

Repetitions
TO EACH SIDE

1	2	3	4	5	6	7
8	9	10	11	12	13	14
15	16	DAY 17 100	DAY 18 100	DAY 19 100	DAY 20 100	DAY 21 100
DAY 22 100	DAY 23 100	DAY 24 100	DAY 25 100	DAY 26 100	DAY 27 100	DAY 28 100
DAY 29 100	DAY 30 100					

Double-Leg Raises

TECHNIQUE

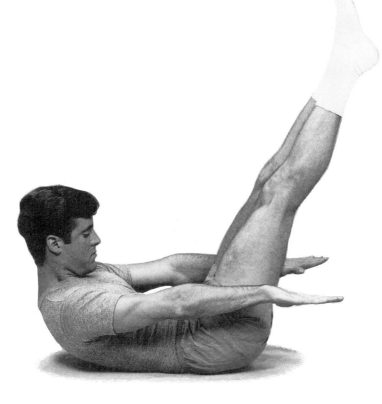

❏ Repeat as in Phase III, very slowly lowering the legs toward the floor, no more than four inches.

NOTE: Now is when you will really start to see fast results, but be sure not to lower your legs so much that your lower back comes into play. Start very slowly, lowering your legs one sixteenth of an inch at a time. Should you feel it in your lower back, come up one sixteenth of an inch at a time. Experiment carefully until you find the position that is comfortable—but challenging—for you.

DON'TS

❏ Do not lift up your legs without bending your knees first.

❏ Do not tense your legs, knees, or toes.

❏ Do not jerk your neck.

❏ Do not tense your neck or shoulders.

❏ Do not move your body back and forth.

Repetitions

1	2	3	4	5	6	7
8	9	10	11	12	13	14
15	16	**DAY 17** **100**	**DAY 18** **100**	**DAY 19** **100**	**DAY 20** **100**	**DAY 21** **100**
DAY 22 **100**	**DAY 23** **100**	**DAY 24** **100**	**DAY 25** **100**	**DAY 26** **100**	**DAY 27** **100**	**DAY 28** **100**
DAY 29 **100**	**DAY 30** **100**					

Both Legs Over

TECHNIQUE

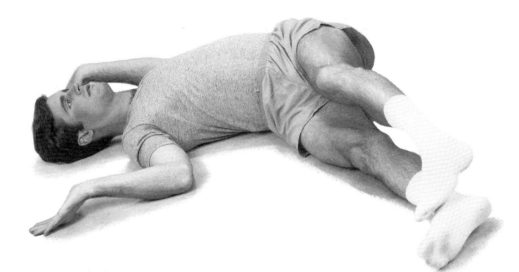

❏ Repeat as in Phase III.

NOTE: *As you become more skilled, you will perform this stretch with greater ease. You will find that you will enter a more relaxed state even quicker. So, a word of warning: If you have somewhere to go or an appointment to keep, be very careful; you can relax so much that you fall asleep!*

DON'TS

❏ Do not tense or jerk your body.

❏ Do not rush through this stretch.

Hold for a count of . . .

TO EACH SIDE

1	2	3	4	5	6	7
8	9	10	11	12	13	14
15	16	DAY 17 **60**	DAY 18 **60**	DAY 19 **60**	DAY 20 **60**	DAY 21 **60**
DAY 22 **60**	DAY 23 **60**	DAY 24 **60**	DAY 25 **60**	DAY 26 **60**	DAY 27 **60**	DAY 28 **60**
DAY 29 **60**	DAY 30 **60**					

Neck to the Side

TECHNIQUE

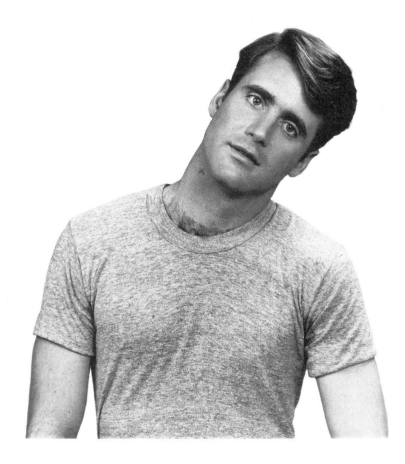

❏ Repeat as in Phase I.

NOTE: Now is when you will become fully aware of the tension in your neck and shoulders and will notice the discomfort it has been causing you. Just remember that you can undo years of tension in just a few minutes a day.

DON'TS

❏ **Do not hunch or tense your shoulders.**

❏ **Do not make any jerky movements.**

Repetitions TO EACH SIDE						
1	2	3	4	5	6	7
8	9	10	11	12	13	14
15	16	DAY 17 1	DAY 18 1	DAY 19 1	DAY 20 1	DAY 21 1
DAY 22 1	DAY 23 1	DAY 24 1	DAY 25 1	DAY 26 1	DAY 27 1	DAY 28 1
DAY 29 1	DAY 30 1					

The Three-Quarter Neck Relaxer

TECHNIQUE

❏ Repeat as in Phase III. If your muscles are very tense, you will feel a stretch between your shoulder blades.

NOTE: Take advantage of this opportunity to be kind to your precious neck! You can perform neck relaxers in so many places: sitting at your desk, watching TV, showering, stuck in a traffic jam . . . do them and see. You'll feel·more alive and so relaxed.

Repetitions
TO EACH SIDE

1	2	3	4	5	6	7
8	9	10	11	12	13	14
15	16	DAY 17 1	DAY 18 1	DAY 19 1	DAY 20 1	DAY 21 1
DAY 22 1	DAY 23 1	DAY 24 1	DAY 25 1	DAY 26 1	DAY 27 1	DAY 28 1
DAY 29 1	DAY 30 1					

DON'TS

❏ Do not force your head down.

❏ Do not tense your shoulders.

LEGS AND INNER THIGHS

Bend and Curl

TECHNIQUE

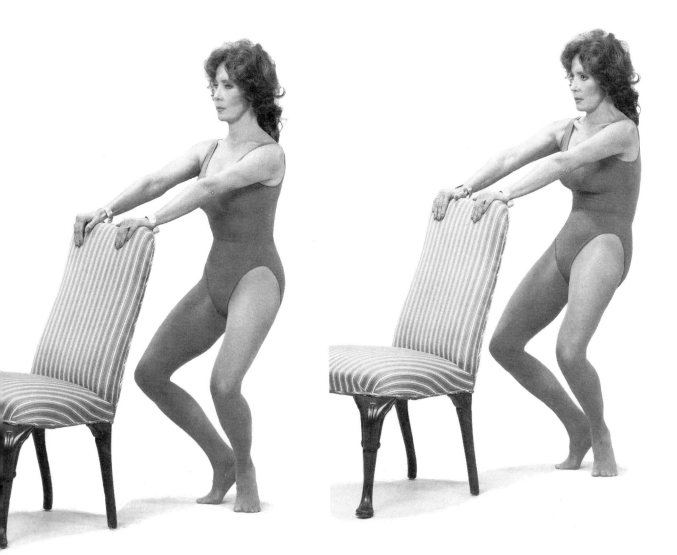

❑ Repeat as in Phase III, lifting your heels as high as you can, so that you are balancing on the balls of your feet, heels together. Go smoothly from one position to the next without holding for the count, as you will be getting double the contraction in this position. If you are able, you may go an inch or two lower, but don't let your buttocks drop lower than your knees, or you will put a terrific strain on your knees.

NOTE: As you gain strength, the tension in your body will begin to disappear. You will also be astonished at how far you are able to curl up your pelvis. As the muscles in your legs, toes, feet, ankles, and calves become stronger, you will be able to go down even lower, working the buttock and stomach muscles even more. As this happens, this exercise will feel easier and easier to do. This exercise also builds strength and flexibility, and you may find that you're able to walk and stand longer without your feet starting to hurt. Suddenly, you'll get that youthful spring back in your step.

DON'TS

❑ **Do not stick out your buttocks or stomach.**

❑ **Do not allow your buttocks to drop lower than your knees.**

❑ **Do not let your heels drop to the floor.**

❑ **Do not tense your shoulders.**

Repetitions

1	2	3	4	5	6	7
8	9	10	11	12	13	14
15	16	DAY 17 7	DAY 18 8	DAY 19 9	DAY 20 10	DAY 21 10
DAY 22 10	DAY 23 10	DAY 24 10	DAY 25 10	DAY 26 10	DAY 27 10	DAY 28 10
DAY 29 10	DAY 30 10					

Plié and Balance

TECHNIQUE

❑ Repeat as in Phase III, lifting your heels even higher so that you are balancing on the balls of your feet, heels together and your feet turned out even further. Lower your body six inches.

NOTE: As you get stronger, you may go down lower than six inches. Just be sure that you do not allow the buttocks to drop lower than your knees, or you will put tremendous pressure on your knees. Before long, you will have the feeling of "floating" like a ballerina!

Repetitions						
1	2	3	4	5	6	7
8	9	10	11	12	13	14
15	16	**DAY 17** 15	**DAY 18** 15	**DAY 19** 16	**DAY 20** 16	**DAY 21** 17
DAY 22 18	**DAY 23** 19	**DAY 24** 20	**DAY 25** 20	**DAY 26** 20	**DAY 27** 20	**DAY 28** 20
DAY 29 20	**DAY 30** 20					

DON'TS

❑ Do not stick out your buttocks or your stomach.

❑ Do not drop your heels, going down or coming up.

❑ Do not tense your shoulders.

Up and Over

TECHNIQUE

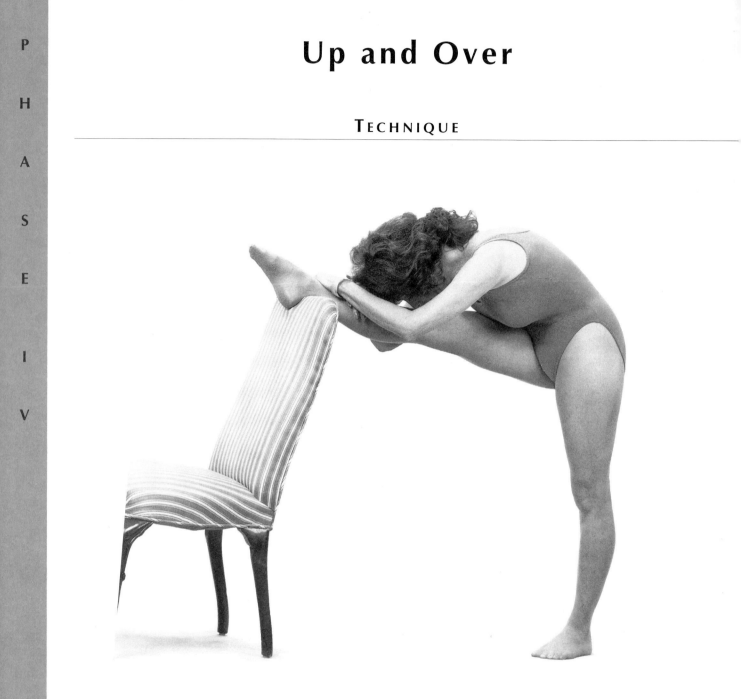

❑ Repeat as in Phase II, straightening your raised leg as much as you can. Your "barre" should now be at its highest level, at least hip high. This time, move your torso up, over, and down the length of your leg as far as you can, continuing to rest your hands on your lower leg. Work both sides.

NOTE: As your muscles stretch, you will be able to bend further and further over your leg. Some people eventually will be able to rest their heads on their legs. Again, if you are very flexible and you need more of a stretch, scoot the standing leg further back from the "barre." You can also get more of a stretch by flexing the raised foot.

 DON'TS

❏ Do not lock either of your knees.

❏ Do not rest your hands on your knees.

❏ Do not make jerking movements with your neck or torso.

❏ Do not force the raised leg straight by pushing the leg or knee down with your hands.

❏ Do not force the raised leg higher than it can easily reach.

❏ Do not put your foot on something so high you cannot keep your balance.

❏ Do not tense your neck and shoulders.

Repetitions
TO EACH SIDE

1	2	3	4	5	6	7
8	9	10	11	12	13	14
15	16	DAY 17 55	DAY 18 55	DAY 19 60	DAY 20 60	DAY 21 60
DAY 22 60	DAY 23 60	DAY 24 60	DAY 25 60	DAY 26 60	DAY 27 60	DAY 28 60
DAY 29 60	DAY 30 60					

Hamstring Stretch

TECHNIQUE

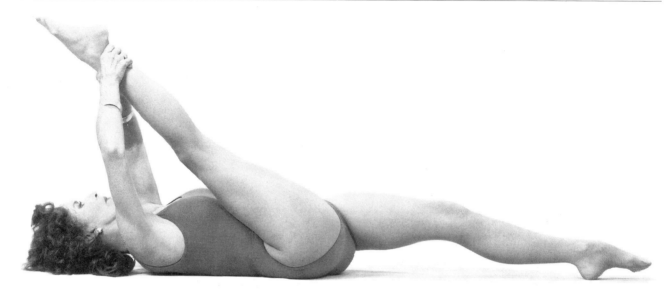

❑ Repeat as in Phase III, continuing to work on straightening your raised leg as much as possible. Once you can do this, *and only then,* concentrate on sliding your extended foot forward until your extended leg is straight out on the floor. Hold for a count of thirty before beginning the repetitions. Work both sides.

NOTE: Once you can perform this exercise with your leg straight out on the floor, you will be stretching the front of the thighs and the difficult-to-reach ilio-psoas. (This is the group of muscles that attach to the front part of the vertebrae in your lower back, deep in the abdomen, and come forward to attach to your femur, or thigh bone. The ilio-psoas allows you to flex the thigh and also to flex the torso without moving your legs.)

DON'TS

❑ **Do not bounce.**

❑ **Do not force the raised leg forward by pulling it.**

❑ **Do not force the raised leg to straighten.**

❑ **Do not tense your neck.**

Repetitions
TO EACH SIDE

1	2	3	4	5	6	7
8	9	10	11	12	13	14
15	16	DAY 17 75	DAY 18 85	DAY 19 95	DAY 20 100	DAY 21 100
DAY 22 100	DAY 23 100	DAY 24 100	DAY 25 100	DAY 26 100	DAY 27 100	DAY 28 100
DAY 29 100	DAY 30 100					

The Standing Stretch

TECHNIQUE

❑ Repeat as in Phase III, trying to curl up your pelvis even more. Gently, try to bring up your bent knee one sixteenth of an inch back—even that much will make an incredible difference that you'll be able to feel. Work both sides.

NOTE: As you continue to do this exercise, not only will you stretch the thigh muscles, but your balance will also improve.

DON'TS

❑ Do not let the foot of the bent leg touch your buttocks.

❑ Do not arch your back or stick out your stomach.

❑ Do not lock your elbows or the knee of the standing leg.

Hold for a count of . . .
TO EACH SIDE

1	2	3	4	5	6	7
8	9	10	11	12	13	14
15	16	DAY 17 50	DAY 18 55	DAY 19 55	DAY 20 60	DAY 21 60
DAY 22 60	DAY 23 60	DAY 24 60	DAY 25 60	DAY 26 60	DAY 27 60	DAY 28 60
DAY 29 60	DAY 30 60					

The Inner-Thigh Tightener

TECHNIQUE

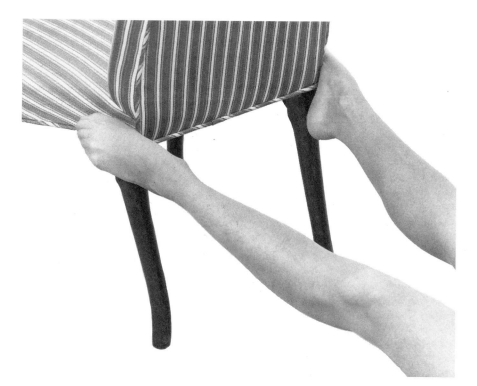

❑ Repeat as in Phase III, continuing to raise your legs one to two inches at a time, until you have reached a maximum of six to eight inches off the floor.

DON'TS

❑ **Do not squeeze and release; hold steadily for the count.**

❑ **Do not tense your shoulders.**

❑ **Do not lock your knees.**

Hold for a count of . . .

1	2	3	4	5	6	7
8	9	10	11	12	13	14
15	16	DAY 17 75	DAY 18 75	DAY 19 75	DAY 20 100	DAY 21 100
DAY 22 100	DAY 23 100	DAY 24 100	DAY 25 100	DAY 26 100	DAY 27 100	DAY 28 100
DAY 29 100	DAY 30 100					

BUTTOCKS, HIPS, AND OUTER THIGHS

Bringing Up the Rear

TECHNIQUE

❏ Repeat as in Phase III, trying to sit straighter and not lean your torso so far to the side. On your working leg, try to keep the foot level with the knee, no higher, to really work the buttock muscles.

NOTE: As your muscles become stronger, you will be able to do this exercise sitting even straighter. Eventually, you won't have to use your hand to roll your hip forward, and your leg will feel light as a feather!

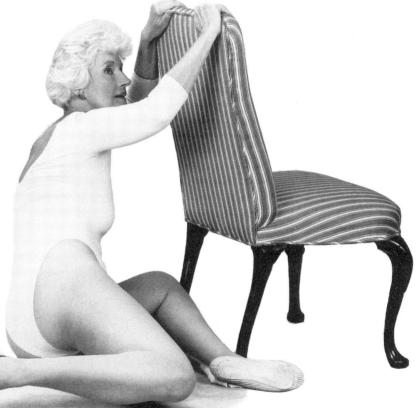

DON'TS

❏ **Do not stick out your buttocks.**

❏ **Do not tense any part of your body, especially your shoulders.**

❏ **Do not push out your stomach.**

❏ **Do not arch your back.**

Repetitions						
TO EACH SIDE						
1	2	3	4	5	6	7
8	9	10	11	12	13	14
15	16	DAY 17 75	DAY 18 85	DAY 19 95	DAY 20 100	DAY 21 100
DAY 22 100	DAY 23 100	DAY 24 100	DAY 25 100	DAY 26 100	DAY 27 100	DAY 28 100
DAY 29 100	DAY 30 100					

Out to the Side

TECHNIQUE

❏ Repeat as in Phase III, rotating your hip even further forward, trying to sit more erect, and keeping your working leg straight. Try to turn your leg so that your knee and toes are pointing into the floor, making the buttock muscles work harder.

NOTE: If you find that with the hip rolled forward, you feel your lower back working, round your upper back and shoulders to straighten your spine.

DON'TS

❏ Do not stick out your stomach.

❏ Do not arch your back.

❏ Do not let your torso lean forward.

❏ Do not lock your knee.

❏ Do not tense your neck or shoulders.

Repetitions

TO EACH SIDE

1	2	3	4	5	6	7
8	9	10	11	12	13	14
15	16	DAY 17 75	DAY 18 85	DAY 19 95	DAY 20 100	DAY 21 100
DAY 22 100	DAY 23 100	DAY 24 100	DAY 25 100	DAY 26 100	DAY 27 100	DAY 28 100
DAY 29 100	DAY 30 100					

Pelvic Circles

TECHNIQUE

❏ Repeat as in Phase III.

NOTE: The stronger you get, the lower you will be able to keep your body and the more you will be able to circle with ease. Soon you will be lifting your body only a few inches off your heels. You will be able to perform this movement smoothly and quickly, taking your hips even further out to the sides and curling up your pelvis even more. With this greater flexibility and range of motion, you will be able to do more repetitions with ease.

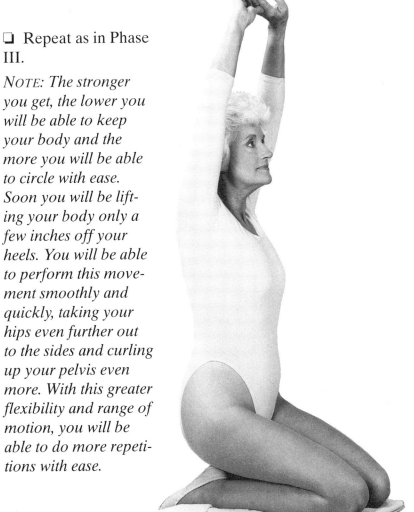
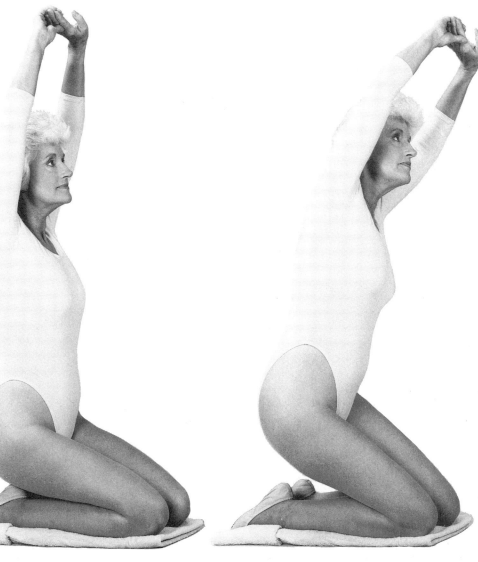

DON'TS

❏ **Do not arch your back.**

❏ **Do not stick out your stomach.**

❏ **Do not try to do too much too fast.**

Repetitions
IN EACH DIRECTION

1	2	3	4	5	6	7
8	9	10	11	12	13	14
15	16	DAY 17 5	DAY 18 5	DAY 19 5	DAY 20 5	DAY 21 5
DAY 22 5	DAY 23 5	DAY 24 5	DAY 25 5	DAY 26 5	DAY 27 5	DAY 28 5
DAY 29 5	DAY 30 5					

The Pelvic Dip

TECHNIQUE

❏ Repeat as in Phase III, lowering your buttocks as if you were going to sit down until you feel them lightly touch your heels. Tighten your buttock muscles and slowly curl up your pelvis. Try to straighten your torso and aim your arms straight up; then return to your starting position, making sure you push your knees together, to make the leg muscles work even more.

NOTE: *As your muscles strengthen, you will continue to improve until this exercise becomes one flowing, graceful motion.*

DON'TS

❏ **Do not arch your back.**

❏ **Do not jerk up your pelvis.**

❏ **Do not let your knees separate.**

Repetitions

1	2	3	4	5	6	7
8	9	10	11	12	13	14
15	16	DAY 17 5	DAY 18 5	DAY 19 5	DAY 20 5	DAY 21 5
DAY 22 5	DAY 23 5	DAY 24 5	DAY 25 5	DAY 26 5	DAY 27 5	DAY 28 5
DAY 29 5	DAY 30 5					

The Front-Thigh Stretch

TECHNIQUE

❑ Repeat as in Phase III. Hold for a count of ten, then curl up your pelvis even more and slowly raise your body half an inch more. In *triple slow motion*, gently lift your pelvis up and down one-sixteenth to one-quarter inch. Release the buttocks and gently return to the original position, sitting on your heels.

NOTE: As you become stronger, you will be able to curl up your pelvis even more, while relaxing your entire body completely.

DON'TS

❑ **Do not arch your back or stick out your stomach.**

❑ **Do not allow your head to drop back.**

❑ **Do not tense your body.**

❑ **Do not hunch your shoulders.**

Repetitions

HOLD FOR A COUNT OF 10

1	2	3	4	5	6	7
8	9	10	11	12	13	14
15	16	DAY 17 **20**	DAY 18 **20**	DAY 19 **20**	DAY 20 **20**	DAY 21 **30**
DAY 22 **30**	DAY 23 **30**	DAY 24 **40**	DAY 25 **40**	DAY 26 **40**	DAY 27 **40**	DAY 28 **40**
DAY 29 **40**	DAY 30 **40**					

The Crossover

TECHNIQUE

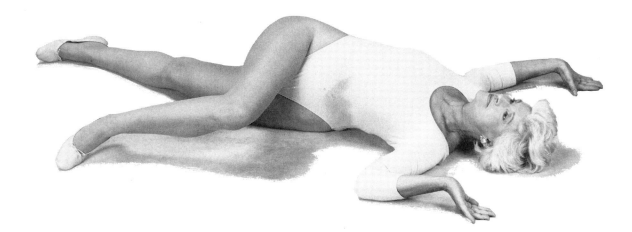

❏ Repeat as in Phase III, bringing your right knee as close to the floor as possible. Keep your left leg straight on the floor in front of you. Work both sides.

NOTE: As your muscles stretch, your flexibility will increase and the bent knee will go lower and lower. You may even be able to touch it to the floor.

DON'TS

❏ **Do not lift your shoulders off the floor.**

❏ **Do not bring your elbows off the floor.**

❏ **Do not turn your head to either side.**

❏ **Do not jerk the bent knee.**

❏ **Do not force the stretch.**

Repetitions
TO EACH SIDE

1	2	3	4	5	6	7
8	9	10	11	12	13	14
15	16	DAY 17 45	DAY 18 50	DAY 19 55	DAY 20 60	DAY 21 60
DAY 22 60	DAY 23 60	DAY 24 60	DAY 25 60	DAY 26 60	DAY 27 60	DAY 28 60
DAY 29 60	DAY 30 60					

Beyond the Countdown

Congratulations! You have now completed the Callanetics Countdown. I'm sure you're more confident about putting on your swimsuit now. You probably also find that you have become calmer and more energized. The calmness can help you enjoy life more. As for the energy Callanetics gives you, don't be surprised at how easy it is to become used to it. It's almost as if you have begun to train your mind as you've trained your body. Stress, anxiety, and tensions start to be relieved, and you are motivated to do more in your life. Fitness takes on a new meaning. It becomes an internal sense of comfort and a feeling of self-worth. For me, this is the most important kind of fitness.

Learning to develop your own unique capabilities instead of being pressured to conform to one standard is what will lead you to make healthy choices in life. Fortunately, the emphasis on "image" in our society is changing. A much wider range of looks is now acceptable, and the need to try to live up to unrealistic expectations is diminishing. Instead, I see more of an emphasis on self-acceptance and wellness, two very important factors that I stress in Callanetics.

Body and mind working for you together is a powerful combination, one that can help you accomplish more than you ever thought possible. More and more studies have shown that exercise can work to prevent certain degenerative problems, like osteoporosis. Some researchers claim that we actually build up immunity to disease when we think positive thoughts and do things that make us feel good. Callanetics gives you this kind of positive reinforcement, and you may find that you want to do more for your body. My recommendation is to listen to this desire and make more time for yourself. Your body is letting you know what it needs.

Maintenance

Once you have finished the Callanetics Countdown, you have several choices. If you have accomplished what you set out to do and are satisfied with the way you look, you can maintain your new shape by practicing your twenty-minute program—by now it probably only takes you ten minutes or so—as little as three times a week. Try to repeat the maximum number of repetitions every time you exercise. You may be so pleased with the results that you decide to work another area of the body.

As you progress, you may find that you want more of a challenge. If that is the case, move on to the regular one-hour Callanetics program found in my first book and video. Once you have mastered that, you can move on to the advanced Super Callanetics program. These are routines that work your entire body, and the results you see and feel will be even more dramatic.

The Winner Within

I've said it before in my previous books, and I'll say it again: Most exercise is boring. If you don't like what you're doing, it won't be fun—and you probably won't see results because you'll be fighting yourself the whole way. You'll find many ways to avoid working, and even you may be surprised at just how creative you can become in your excuses. Even though Callanetics makes me feel so wonderful, there are times when even I just don't want to exercise. I try to remember just how good my body feels and, on most days, once I start I'm fine. But on those days when nothing seems to work, I devise a little fantasy to get myself motivated. I just imagine myself in a situation that requires as much physical and mental strength as I can muster. My favorite is a fencing duel in which I must defend my honor and literally fight for my life. I always embellish it with lots of "Walter Mitty" detail, and it works every time. I suggest you try it, too.

The important thing is to try to see what you can do. I am convinced there is a winner in everyone. But only you know what your individual potential is, and only you can decide how much of it you are going to discover. I always remind myself of the old story about the bumblebee. Aerodynamically, the bumblebee is not supposed to be able to fly, because its body weight is too heavy for its wingspan. But it does fly. And all because it doesn't know it can't. So give yourself a chance, and when you think (or someone else tells you) that something is impossible for you, just remember the bumblebee.

About the Author

Callan Pinckney was raised in Savannah, Georgia. She trained in classical ballet for twelve years and has studied other forms of dance, movement, and exercise. She had to restore her own body to health when, after an eleven-year backpacking odyssey around the world, the rigors of travel, combined with a congenital back defect, led to physical collapse. This was the beginning of Callanetics. She is the author of *Callanetics* and *Callanetics for Your Back*. She divides her time between New York City and Savannah.

Notes

Notes

Notes

PHASE III

Notes